TEAM

**Trauma Evaluation
and Management**

The Subcommittee on ATLS® to the American College of Surgeons Committee on Trauma, as contributing authors to the TEAM course, have taken care that the doses of drugs and recommendations for treatment contained herein are correct and compatible with the standards generally accepted at the time of publication. However, as new research and clinical experience broaden our knowledge, changes in treatment and drug therapy may become necessary or appropriate. Readers and participants of this course are advised to check the most current product information provided by the manufacturer of each drug to be administered to verify the recommended dose, the method and duration of administration, and contraindications. It is the responsibility of the licensed practitioner to be informed in all aspects of patient care and determine the best treatment for each individual patient. The American College of Surgeons, its Committee on Trauma, the Subcommittee on ATLS, and contributing authors disclaim any liability, loss, or damage incurred as a consequence, directly or indirectly, of the use and application of any of the content of this third edition of the TEAM program.

Third Edition

Table of Contents

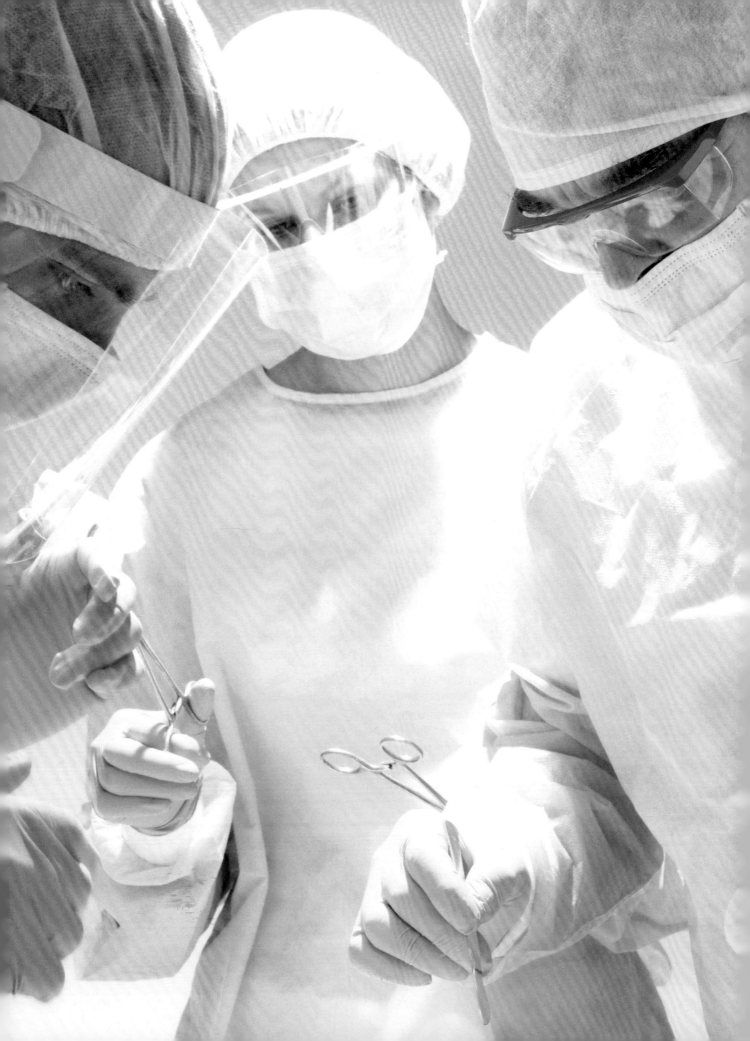

CORE CONTENT

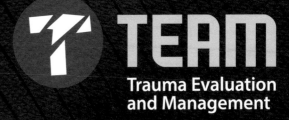

EMERGENCY

CLEARANCE 8'-2"

STOP HERE
<< ENTRANCE

Trauma Evaluation and Management Program

Trauma Evaluation and Management (TEAM): Early Care of the Injured Patient— a program for medical students and multidisciplinary team members—is based on the *ATLS Course for Doctors*.

SLIDE 1

Program Goals

This Trauma Evaluation and Management (TEAM) Program provides the program participant with an overview of the purpose and concepts of immediate management of the injured patient and a basic understanding of the fundamental principles of trauma care, including:

SLIDE 2

1. Rapid, accurate, and physiologic assessment of the patient's condition.
2. Resuscitation, stabilization, and monitoring of the patient, according to priority.
3. Preparation for the patient's interhospital transfer, if the patient's needs exceed the facility's capabilities.
4. Introduction of concepts of injury prevention strategies.

Program Objectives

Upon completion of this program, the participant will be able to describe the principles of early care in the multiply injured patient. Specifically, the participant will be able to:

SLIDE 3, 4

1. Describe the fundamental principles of initial assessment and management.
2. Identify the correct sequence of priorities used in assessing the multiply injured patient.
3. Describe guidelines and techniques used in the initial resuscitation and definitive-care phases when treating the multiply injured patient.
4. Identify how the patient's medical history and the mechanism of injury contribute to the identification of injuries.
5. Identify the concepts related to teamwork in caring for the injured patient.
6. Describe strategies for injury prevention.

Notes:

Introduction

The purpose of the TEAM Program is to orient participants to the initial evaluation and early management of the trauma patient. In general, the concepts presented in these materials are derived from the *Advanced Trauma Life Support (ATLS) Course for Doctors*, sponsored by the American College of Surgeons. The ATLS Course provides further details, essential information, and skills that should be applied to the identification and treatment of life-threatening injuries by the first responding doctor.

The ATLS Student Course provides further education in the essential information and skills the first responding doctors should apply to the identification and treatment of life-threatening or potentially life-threatening injuries. Medical students are permitted to take the ATLS Student Course in their final year of medical school and receive a document attesting to their successful completion upon graduation from medical school.

Notes:

The Need

Global trauma-related dollar costs exceed $500 billion annually. These costs are much higher if we consider lost wages, medical expenses, insurance administration costs, property damage, fire loss, employer costs, and indirect loss from work-related injuries. Yet with these staggering costs, less than 4 cents of each federal research dollar is expended on trauma research in the United States. As monumental as these data are, the true cost to society can be measured only when it is realized that trauma strikes down its youngest and potentially most productive members. As tragic as is any "accidental" death, the loss of life in the early years is the most tragic of all. Research dollars spent on communicable diseases—for example, poliomyelitis and diphtheria—have nearly eliminated these diseases in the United States. Amazingly, the disease of trauma has not captured the public attention in the same way.

SLIDE 5

Injury deaths worldwide have been estimated at more than 5 million in 2000. By 2020, injury may advance to become the second or third leading cause of death in all age groups. Figure 1 demonstrates conclusively that the problem of injury is a significant world health issue. (See Figure 1, Death Rates from Injury per 100,000 Population.) Injury does not discriminate based on age, race, sex, or economic status. It is the leading cause of death in persons aged one through 44 years in most developed countries and is assuming a more prominent position in lower-income nations as infectious diseases are eradicated.

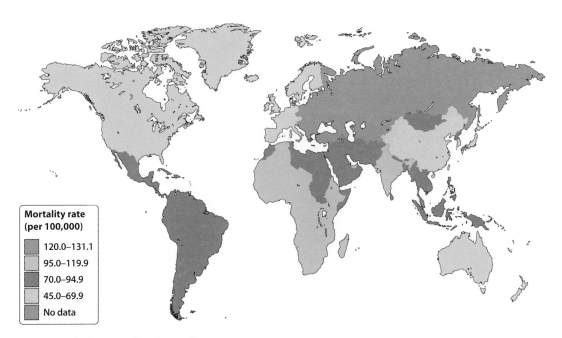

**Mortality rate
(per 100,000)**

- 120.0–131.1
- 95.0–119.9
- 70.0–94.9
- 45.0–69.9
- No data

Figure 1 Global Injury-Related Mortality.
Reproduced with permission from *The Injury Chart Book: A Graphical Overview of the Global Burden of Injuries*. Geneva: World Health Organization Department of Injuries and Violence Prevention, Noncommunicable Diseases and Mental Health Cluster; 2002.

Motor vehicle crashes (MVCs) account for the majority of injuries and deaths worldwide. The incidence of fatal mechanisms of injury varies from country to country. For example, the rate for vehicular mortality is highest in New Zealand, being nearly 2.5 times the rate in the Bahamas and the United Kingdom. Figure 2 demonstrates the global distribution of injury mortality by cause. Falls, drownings, and burns generally follow traffic crashes as leading injury mechanisms.

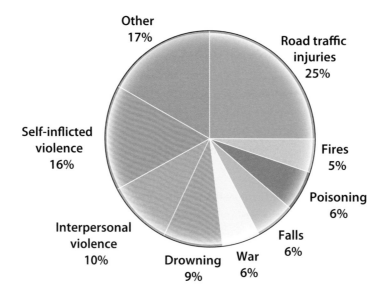

Figure 2 Distribution of Global Injury Mortality by Cause.
Reproduced with permission from *The Injury Chart Book: A Graphical Overview of the Global Burden of Injuries.* Geneva: World Health Organization Department of Injuries and Violence Prevention, Noncommunicable Diseases and Mental Health Cluster; 2002.

Deaths from firearms are a particular problem in the United States, Norway, Israel, and France. The mortality rate in the United States from guns approaches the rate due to vehicular trauma for the age group of 15 to 24 years: 13.7 versus 16.2 per 100,000 population. The availability of weapons in the United States, compared with other nations of the world, may be a contributing factor to this problem. The mortality rate from firearms is so low in 25 of the 39 countries that the rates are not reported.

Data reflecting the rates of disability from injury in the United States and Portugal show that permanent disability dwarfs the mortality rate by 3 to 1. In 1998, more than 19.4 million disabling injuries occurred in the United States: one every two seconds. For each vehicular fatality in Portugal in 1996, 31 people sustained some disability.

More than 60 million injuries occur in the United States each year resulting in an average of 36.8 million visits to emergency centers. This figure represents 40 percent of all emergency department visits. Fifty-four percent of these visits are by children aged five to 14 years. For every injury death there are 19 hospital admissions, 233 emergency department visits, and 450 office-based doctor visits for medical attention related to injury. These data indicate that care for the injured patient consumes a significant proportion of the health care resources of any nation.

Injury is a disease. It has a host (the patient), and it has a vector of transmission (motor vehicle, firearm, etc). Great strides have been made in the eradication of infectious diseases. Cancer and heart disease prevention and treatment have extended the life expectancy of the populations in developed countries. Compared with other diseases, only a small amount of money and effort has been expended to combat injury, a disease that affects the potentially most productive members of any society and its most valuable national resource, the children. The economic impact is staggering considering the lost wages, medical expenses, administration costs, property damage, and indirect costs. It would be so simple to apply recognized injury prevention strategies—be they primary (avoidance, achieved through education), secondary (attenuation, attained through engineering), or tertiary (amelioration, acquired through emergency medical and trauma care)—which have been shown to decrease the overall burden and cost of injury by as much as 50% to 80% in several studies. Sadly, they have not been implemented to the degree necessary to make a difference in trauma morbidity and mortality.

Many significant changes have improved the care of the injured patient since the first edition of the ATLS Course appeared in 1980. Nevertheless, trauma remains the leading cause of death in the first 4 decades of life (ages one through 44 years), surpassed only by cancer and atherosclerosis as the major causes of death in all age groups. As great as the death rate from injury is—approximately 161,296[1] deaths occur annually in the United States—permanent disability from injury dwarfs the mortality by 3 to 1. The societal cost is staggering, as is the amount of human suffering. The need for improved methods of caring for injured patients is vitally important. The need for the program, and for sustained aggressive efforts to prevent injuries, is as great now as it has ever been. Unfortunately, public awareness has not translated into public utilization and acceptance (for example, use of seat belts and helmets). Until the public utilizes these preventative methods and modalities, training in trauma evaluation and management will be even more necessary.

[1]National Center for Injury Prevention and Control, 2002 United States, All Injury Deaths.

Notes:

Trimodal Death Distribution

The frequency of deaths after injury follows a trimodal distribution. (See Figure 3, Trimodal Death Distribution.) The **first peak** of this distribution occurs within seconds to minutes after injury. During this early period, deaths generally result from lacerations of the brain, brain stem, high spinal cord, heart, aorta, and other large blood vessels. Very few of these patients can be salvaged due to the severity of their injuries. Salvage after injury during this peak can be achieved only in certain large urban areas where rapid prehospital care and transport are available. Only prevention can significantly reduce this peak of traumatic deaths.

SLIDE 6

The **second peak** occurs within minutes to several hours following injury. The TEAM Program focuses primarily on this period. Deaths occurring during this period are usually due to subdural and epidural hematomas, hemopneumothorax, ruptured spleen, lacerations of the liver, pelvic fractures, and/or other multiple injuries associated with significant blood loss. The "first hour" of care after injury focuses on rapid assessment and resuscitation, which are the hallmarks of trauma evaluation and management. The concept of the "golden hour" emphasizes the **urgency** of successful management in order to optimize outcome of the injured patient and is not intended to imply a "fixed" time period of 60 minutes.

In the **third peak**, occurring several days to weeks after the initial injury, death is most often due to sepsis and multiple organ system failure. Care provided during each of the preceding time periods affects outcome during this stage. Thus, the first and every subsequent individual caring for the injured patient have a direct effect on long-term outcome.

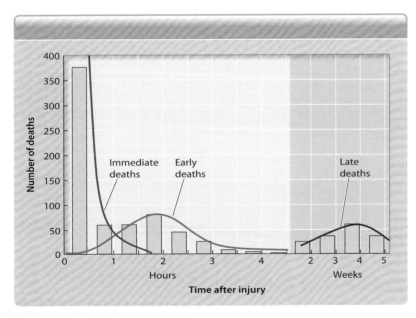

Figure 3 Trimodal Death Distribution
Modified with permission from Trunkey DD: *Scientific American* 1989. 3;249;28-35.

Notes:

The Concept

The concept behind trauma evaluation and management is simple. The approach to the injured patient is not the same as that for a patient with a previously undiagnosed medical condition, that is, an extensive history including past medical history, a physical examination starting at the top of the head and progressing down the body, and finally the development of a differential diagnosis and a list of adjuncts to confirm a diagnosis. This approach is quite adequate for a patient with diabetes mellitus or even many acute surgical illnesses. However, it does not satisfy the needs of the patient suffering life-threatening injury.

There are six underlying precepts of trauma evaluation and management. The most important of these precepts is to treat the greatest threat to life first. Second, the lack of a definitive diagnosis should never impede the application of an indicated treatment, and a detailed history is not essential to begin the evaluation of an acutely injured patient. Third is the need for a physiologic approach to the evaluation and treatment of the injured. The fourth is that injury kills in certain reproducible time frames. Thus, time is of the essence. The fifth is to do no further harm. The sixth is teamwork. Teamwork (multidisciplinary team members) is required for TEAM to succeed.

SLIDE 7

Notes:

Physiologic Approach

The physiologic approach to the evaluation and treatment of the injured patient is based on the principle that the airway, breathing, and circulation constitute an integrated system aimed at preserving cell function by maintaining oxygen delivery to these cells. Core organs (for example, the brain) require a continuous supply of oxygen and nutrients for optimal function. Because of the sequential nature of oxygen delivery, a patent airway and adequate breathing are necessary before the circulation can deliver oxygen. Therefore, the loss of an airway or ability to breathe kills more quickly than does diminished circulating blood volume. The presence of neurologic disability or altered mental status, particularly if caused by an expanding intracranial mass lesion, is the next most lethal problem.

SLIDE 8

The mnemonic "ABCDE" defines the specific, ordered evaluations and interventions that should be followed in all injured patients:

A **A**irway maintenance with cervical-spine protection

B **B**reathing and ventilation with life-threatening chest injury management

C **C**irculation with hemorrhage control

D **D**isability or neurologic status with intracranial mass lesion recognition

E **E**xposure/**E**nvironment with maintenance of normal body temperature

Notes:

Primary Survey

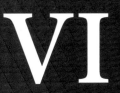

Initial assessment and management are optimally performed in a set sequence. The primary survey, **conducted simultaneously with resuscitation**, consists of a rapid, systematic evaluation of the airway, breathing, circulation, disability, and exposure/environment, treating life-threatening conditions as they are discovered. Adjuncts, such as urinary and gastric catheters, vital signs, monitoring devices, and chest and pelvic X-rays facilitate the process of discovery.

SLIDE 9

The secondary survey consists of a focused injury history and detailed physical examination, **conducted simultaneously with reassessment of the patient's ABCDEs**, designed to pinpoint the exact nature of the injuries. Adjuncts—for example, laboratory tests and special X-ray and/or diagnostic studies—help to establish a definitive diagnosis.

The primary and secondary surveys should be repeated frequently to identify any deterioration in the patient's status. Any necessary treatment should be initiated at the time an adverse change is identified. Continuous reevaluation and optimal stabilization complete the initial assessment and management process even while the patient is being prepared for transfer to the operating room, the intensive care unit, or another facility, as needed.

This sequence is presented as an overview of a linear or longitudinal progression of events. **In the actual clinical situation, many of these activities occur in parallel or simultaneously** if additional personnel are available. The linear or longitudinal progression allows the doctor an opportunity to mentally review the progress of an actual trauma resuscitation while maintaining an order of priority related to the degree of life threat.

SLIDE 10

Notes:

"TEAM" Work and Teamwork VII

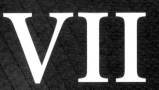

Trauma evaluation and management (TEAM) occur sequentially based on essential physiologic priorities (ABCDs)—airway leads to breathing, which leads to circulation. Although the early care of the injured patient presented in the TEAM Program may be provided by a single doctor, there often are multiple doctors, nurses, and allied health professionals available to assist in the resuscitation of the injured patient. Accordingly, the patient's airway, breathing, and circulation may be evaluated and managed simultaneously, rather than sequentially. In such circumstances, teamwork is required for TEAM work to succeed.

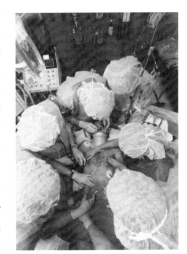

"TEAM" also is an acronym for "**T**ogether **E**veryone **A**chieves **M**ore." In ideal trauma systems, trauma care is delivered by a multidisciplinary team, following the same physiologic priorities presented in the TEAM Program, yet more in parallel with another than in a series of critical interventions. The team remains focused on the early care of the injured patient and synchronizes activities to produce safe and effective patient care. Teamwork also reduces missed injuries and improves patient outcome by providing a structure for comprehensive evaluation and timely management in a sometimes hectic setting.

Composition of the multidisciplinary team may vary depending on available personnel and expertise. The team described here includes the team leader (trauma doctor), airway manager (trauma doctor, emergency medicine doctor, anesthesiologist, nurse anesthetist, or respiratory therapist), nurse, and assistants. Each member has specific roles and responsibilities, which must be known and practiced by every member of the team, according to the diagram in Figure 3, Trauma Team.

A. The team leader manages the primary and secondary surveys, ensuring linkage between evaluation and management.

B. The airway manager focuses on providing and maintaining a patent airway, ventilation, and oxygenation.

C. The nurse collects specific data, for example, vital signs, as needed for trauma evaluation and management, and monitors activity in the resuscitation room.

D. The assistants perform specific tasks, such as removing the patient's clothing, inserting intravenous catheters, administering fluids, and obtaining blood and urinary specimens.

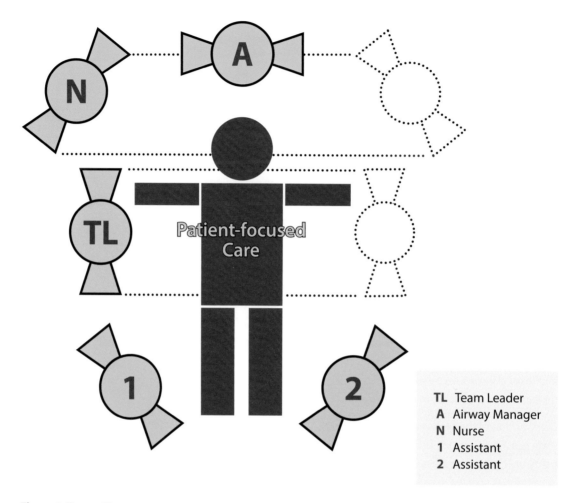

TL	Team Leader
A	Airway Manager
N	Nurse
1	Assistant
2	Assistant

Figure 4 Trauma Team.
Illustration used with permission from LTC(P) John Armstrong and MAJ Brad West, US Army.

The role of the team leader and airway manager may be the combined responsibility of one individual in the absence of multiple providers with the requisite skills for trauma resuscitation. Medical students, residents, emergency medical technicians, paramedics, radiology personnel, blood bank personnel, and subspecialty surgeons also are important members of the team across the care continuum.

The multidisciplinary trauma team that plans and practices becomes more efficient and avoids unfocused and redundant efforts. This efficiency further leads to error reduction and improved patient safety.

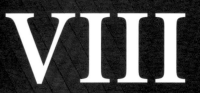

Preparation for the trauma patient occurs in two different clinical settings. First, during the prehospital phase, all events must be coordinated with the doctors at the receiving hospital. Second, during the inhospital phase, preparations must be made to rapidly facilitate the resuscitation of the trauma patient.

A. Prehospital Phase

SLIDE 12

Coordination with the prehospital agency and personnel can greatly expedite the treatment in the field. The prehospital system should be set up such that the receiving hospital is notified before the prehospital personnel transport the patient from the scene. This allows mobilization of the hospital's Trauma Team members so that all necessary personnel and resources are present in the emergency department at the time of the patient's arrival. Emphasis in the prehospital phase should be placed on airway maintenance, support of breathing, control of external bleeding and shock, immobilization of the patient, and immediate transport to the **closest appropriate facility**, preferably a verified trauma center. Every effort should be made to minimize scene time. (See Appendix 2, Prehospital Triage Decision Scheme.) Emphasis also should be placed on obtaining and reporting information needed for triage at the hospital, for example, time of injury, events related to the injury, and patient history. The mechanisms of injury may suggest the degree of injury as well as specific injuries for which the patient must be evaluated.

The use of prehospital care protocols and online medical direction can facilitate and improve care initiated in the field. Periodic multidisciplinary review of the care provided through quality assurance/improvement activities is essential.

B. Inhospital Phase

SLIDE 13

Advanced planning for the trauma patient's arrival is essential. Ideally, a resuscitation area should be available for trauma patients. Proper airway equipment (laryngoscopes, endotracheal tubes, and so on) should be organized, tested, and strategically placed where it is immediately accessible. Warmed intravenous crystalloid solutions (for example, Ringer's lactate) should be available and ready for infusion when the patient arrives. Appropriate monitoring capabilities should be immediately available. A method to summon extra medical assistance should be in place. A means to ensure prompt response by laboratory and radiology personnel is necessary. Transfer agreements with a verified trauma center should be preestablished and operational. Periodic review of the care through the quality improvement process is an essential component of the hospital's trauma program.

SLIDE 14

All personnel who have contact with the patient must be protected from communicable diseases. Most prominent among these diseases are hepatitis and human immunodeficiency virus (HIV) infection. The Centers for Disease Control and Prevention (CDC) and other health agencies strongly recommend the use of standard precautions (for example, cap, face mask, eye protection, water-impervious gown/apron, leggings, and gloves) when coming in contact with body fluids. The ACS Committee on Trauma considers these to be minimum precautions for protection of all health care providers. This also is an Occupational Safety and Health Administration (OSHA) requirement in the United States.

Notes:

Triage

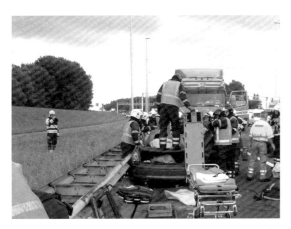

Triage is the treatment prioritization of multiple patients based on the need for treatment and the available resources to provide that treatment. Treatment is rendered based on the ABC priorities (**A**irway with cervical spine protection, **B**reathing with life-threatening chest injury management, and **C**irculation with hemorrhage control), as outlined later in this document. Other factors considered in the triage process are severity of injuries; salvageability; and available resources, including time, personnel, and operating rooms.

Triage takes place in the field (primary triage) and at the medical facility to which patients are to be transported (secondary triage). It is the responsibility of the prehospital personnel and their medical director to see that the appropriate patients arrive at the appropriate hospital. It is inappropriate for prehospital personnel to deliver a severely traumatized patient to a nontrauma center hospital if a trauma center is available. (See Appendix 2, Prehospital Triage Decision Scheme.) Prehospital trauma scoring is helpful in identifying those severely injured patients who should be transported to a trauma center. (See Appendix 3, Revised and Pediatric Trauma Scores.) Two types of triage situations usually exist.

A. Multiple Casualty Incidents

The number of patients and the severity of their injuries do **not** exceed the ability of the facility to render care. In this situation, patients whose survival is in doubt because of the severity of their injuries may need to be treated last. This allows available resources to be used in a manner that does the most good for the largest number of injured patients.

B. Mass Casualty Incidents

The number of patients and the severity of their injuries exceed the capability of the facility and staff. In this situation, those patients with the greatest chance of survival, and requiring the least expenditure of time, equipment, supplies, and personnel, are managed first.

Notes:

Primary Survey

Patients are assessed and their treatment priorities established based on the degree of life threat posed by their injuries, their vital signs, and the injury mechanism. These priorities are the same for all injured patients, including adult, pediatric, pregnant, and geriatric patients. In the severely injured patient, logical sequential treatment priorities must be established based on overall patient assessment. The patient's vital functions must be assessed quickly and efficiently. Patient management must consist of a rapid primary evaluation, resuscitation of vital functions, a more detailed secondary assessment, and finally, the initiation of definitive care. This process constitutes the ABCDEs of trauma care and identifies life-threatening conditions by adhering to this sequence:

A **A**irway maintenance with cervical spine protection

SLIDES 16, 17

B **B**reathing with life-threatening chest injury management

C **C**irculation with hemorrhage control

D **D**isability: Brief neurologic examination with intracranial mass lesion recognition

E **E**xposure/**E**nvironmental with maintenance of normal body temperature

During the primary survey, life-threatening conditions are identified and management is instituted **simultaneously**. The prioritized assessment and management procedures reviewed in this chapter are identified as sequential steps in order of importance for the purpose of clarity, and to provide a protocol that a "team leader" should follow when alone. When other personnel are available, these steps are frequently accomplished simultaneously.

Quick Assessment

Within 10 seconds it is possible to asses the critical nature of injuries sustained by the trauma patient. This is done by:

SLIDES 18, 19

(a) Identifying yourself

(b) Asking patient his/her name

(c) Asking the patient what happened

An appropriate response suggests that the patient has:

(a) A patent airway

(b) Sufficient air reserve to permit speech

(c) Sufficient perfusion to preserve cerebration

(d) Clear sensorium

An inappropriate response suggests urgent problems affecting A, B, C, or D requiring urgent intervention(s).

Special Considerations

Pediatric patient

SLIDES 20, 21, 22

Trauma is the leading cause of death in the **pediatric patient**. Anatomic and physiologic differences from the adult include both developmentally immature features of the child and a vigorous compensatory response to major trauma, which is relatively short-lived due to limited compensatory reserves. However, priorities for the care of the pediatric patient are the same as for adults. In managing the airway and ventilation, it must be remembered that the larynx is cephalad and anterior and that the trachea is relatively short, making intubation more difficult. The mobile mediastinum and pliable chest wall result in greater susceptibility to tension pneumothorax and pulmonary contusions. Although volume resuscitation is less often needed in the pediatric trauma patient because head injuries are more common than torso injuries, intraosseous vascular access is more likely to be required in the pediatric trauma patient. The response to volume loss, vital signs, and urinary output also are dependent on the size of the child. In head trauma, vomiting and seizures are common with minor head injury. Diffuse brain swelling is more common with major head injury, while in infants the open fontanelles may minimize increases in intracranial pressure. Although the quantities of blood, fluids, and medications; the size of the child; the degree and rapidity of heat loss; and injury patterns may differ, assessment and management priorities are identical. Outcome depends on early aggressive care.

Pregnant patient

SLIDES 23, 24

Priorities for the care of the **pregnant woman** are similar to those for the nonpregnant patient, but the anatomic and physiologic changes of pregnancy may modify the patient's response to injury. Variations in position of the uterus with gestational age, the physiologic anemia resulting from increases in plasma volume relative to red blood cell mass, the characteristic hyperventilation with a low arterial PCO_2, decreased gastric emptying, the supine hypotension resulting from compression of the vena cava by the gravid uterus, the risk of isoimmunization in the Rh-negative mother, and the extreme sensitivity of the placental circulation to maternal hypovolemia are some of the important considerations in the approach to managing the injured pregnant patient. Early recognition of pregnancy by appropriate history, palpation of the abdomen for a gravid uterus, and laboratory testing for human chorionic gonadotropin, along with early fetal assessment, is important for maternal and fetal survival. However, the first priority is maternal resuscitation.

Geriatric patient

Trauma is the fifth most common cause of death in the **geriatric patient**. With increasing age, cardiovascular disease and cancer overtake injury as the leading causes of death. Interestingly, the risk of death for any given injury at the lower and moderate injury severity score (ISS) levels is greater for the elderly man than for the elderly woman. The aging process diminishes the physiologic reserve of the elderly trauma patient. Chronic cardiac, respiratory, and metabolic disease may reduce the ability of the geriatric patient to compensate for the physiologic stress imposed by injury the way younger patients are able to do. Comorbidities, such as diabetes, congestive heart failure, coronary artery disease, restrictive and obstructive pulmonary disease, coagulopathy, liver disease, and peripheral vascular disease are more common and adversely affect outcome following injury to the older patient. The chronic use of medications may alter the usual physiologic response to injury. The narrow therapeutic window frequently leads to overresuscitation or underresuscitation in this patient population, and early invasive monitoring is frequently a valuable adjunct to management. Despite these facts, the majority of elderly trauma patients will recover and return to their preinjury level of independent activity if appropriately managed. Prompt aggressive resuscitation and the early recognition of preexisting medical conditions and medication use can improve the survival of this group.

SLIDE 25

A. **Airway Maintenance with Cervical Spine Protection**

Every effort should be made to promptly identify airway compromise and secure a patent airway. Upon initial evaluation of the trauma patient, the airway should be assessed first to ascertain patency. This rapid assessment for signs of airway obstruction should include inspection for foreign bodies and facial, mandibular, or tracheal/laryngeal fractures that may result in airway obstruction.

1. Airway maintenance

SLIDE 26

Airway obstruction is identified and managed during the primary survey. Airway obstruction must be immediately recognized and promptly corrected. Snoring, gurgling, stridor, hoarseness, and rocking chest wall motions are indicative of airway obstruction. Equally important is the recognition of the potential for progressive airway loss. Frequent reevaluation of airway security is essential to identify the patient who is losing the ability to maintain an adequate airway.

SLIDE 27

Measures to establish a patent airway should be instituted while protecting the cervical spine. Initially, simple measures such as the chin lift or modified jaw thrust maneuver may achieve this task. Airway suctioning is then performed as necessary to clear excessive secretions, using a large-caliber suction catheter. Particulate matter is removed, if present, using a finger-sweep or forceps. Airway adjuncts (for example, oropharyngeal airway) may be necessary to maintain airway patency in patients who are unconscious and have lost their gag reflex.

If the patient is able to communicate verbally, the airway is not likely to be in immediate jeopardy; however, repeated assessment of airway patency is prudent, especially in patients with respiratory compromise or maxillofacial injury. If the patient is unable to maintain spontaneous respiration or patency of the airway, then a definitive airway is indicated. A definitive airway is defined as a secured tube in the trachea with the cuff inflated and the tube connected to some form of oxygen-enriched assisted ventilation. A definitive airway usually is obtained via the orotracheal route, with other techniques being applied as indicated.

In the pediatric age group, uncuffed tubes may be used. Severe head-injury patients with an altered level of consciousness or a Glasgow Coma Scale (GCS) Score of eight or less usually require the placement of a definitive airway. The finding of nonpurposeful motor responses strongly suggests the need for definitive airway management. Management of the pediatric airway requires a knowledge of the unique anatomic features of the position and size of the larynx in children, as well as special equipment.

2. Cervical spine protection

While assessing and managing the patient's airway, great care should be taken to prevent excessive movement of the cervical spine. The patient's head and neck should not be hyperextended, hyperflexed, or rotated to establish and maintain the airway. Based on the history of the trauma incident, the loss of stability of the cervical spine should be suspected. Neurologic examination alone does not exclude a cervical spine injury. Protection of the patient's spinal cord with manual, inline immobilization followed by the application of appropriate immobilization devices should be accomplished. If immobilizing devices must be removed temporarily, the neutral position of the patient's head and neck should be reinstituted with manual, inline immobilization by one member of the trauma team. Immobilization devices used to protect the patient's spinal cord should be left in place until cervical spine injury is excluded. **Protection of the spine and spinal cord is the important management principle.** Cervical spine X-rays or CT Scan may be obtained to confirm or exclude injury once immediate or potentially life-threatening conditions have been addressed. **Remember: Assume a cervical spine injury in any patient with multisystem trauma, especially with an altered level of consciousness or a blunt injury above the clavicle.**

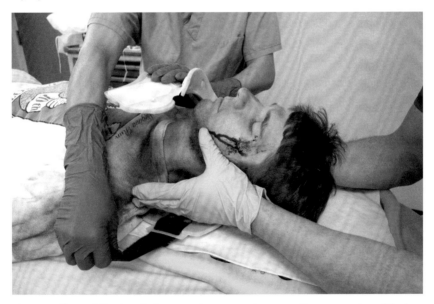

Figure 5 If immobilization devices must be removed temporarily, one member of the trauma team should manually stabilize the patient's head and neck using inline immobilization techniques.

B. Breathing with Life-threatening Chest Injury Management

The initial step in managing respiratory failure in the injured patient is to recognize its presence. No laboratory tests diagnose respiratory failure. The initial diagnosis is based on clinical appreciation of the presence of inadequate or ineffective ventilation and oxygenation.

1. Respiratory mechanics and gas exchange

SLIDE 28

Airway patency alone does not assure adequate ventilation. Adequate gas exchange is required to maximize oxygenation and carbon dioxide elimination. Ventilation requires adequate function of the lungs, chest wall, and diaphragm. Each component must be examined and evaluated rapidly.

The patient's chest should be exposed to adequately assess chest wall excursion. Auscultation should be performed to assure gas flow in the lungs. Adequacy of ventilation should be assessed through observation of chest wall mechanics, that is, accessory muscle use and ventilatory rate. Percussion may suggest the presence of air or blood in the chest. Visual inspection and palpation may detect injuries to the chest wall that may compromise ventilation.

2. Immediately life-threatening chest injuries

SLIDE 29

Immediately life-threatening chest injuries must be recognized and managed during the primary survey. Injuries that may acutely impair ventilation are tension pneumothorax, flail chest with pulmonary contusion, massive hemothorax, and open pneumothorax. These injuries should be identified in the primary survey. Simple pneumo- or hemothorax, fractured ribs, and pulmonary contusion may compromise ventilation to a lesser degree and are usually identified in the secondary survey.

Tension and open pneumothorax are identified and controlled in the primary survey. A tension pneumothorax compromises ventilation and circulation dramatically and acutely and is diagnosed clinically. If suspected, needle decompression should be accomplished immediately, followed later by chest tube insertion. **Remember, a tension pneumothorax is a clinical diagnosis and not a radiologic diagnosis.** An open pneumothorax also compromises ventilation dramatically and acutely, and if suspected, the chest wall defect should be treated immediately with an occlusive dressing followed by a chest tube insertion. (See Appendix 1, Glossary of Frequently Confused Terms.)

C. Circulation with Hemorrhage Control

SLIDE 30

Shock in the trauma patient may be hemorrhagic or nonhemorrhagic. Of these, hemorrhage is the most common cause of shock in the injured patient and is the predominant cause of postinjury deaths that are preventable by rapid treatment in the hospital setting. The trauma patient in shock should therefore be considered to be in hemorrhagic shock until proven otherwise. **Hemorrhage must therefore be identified and stopped as soon as possible.** External bleeding is controlled by direct pressure. Internal hemorrhage may require operative intervention. Internal sources of hemorrhage may be the chest, abdomen, pelvis, or retroperitoneum. The combination of history, physical examination, and chest X ray with focused assessment sonography in trauma (FAST) and X rays of the pelvis frequently identify the source of internal hemorrhage. In the patient who is not hemodynamically compromised, CT scan also is very helpful and more specific than FAST in identifying the source of hemorrhage.

SLIDE 31

If the shock is nonhemorrhagic, then obstructive causes of shock (for example, tension pneumothorax and cardiac tamponade), must be considered. Hypotension with bradycardia should suggest the presence of neurogenic shock. Although septic shock occurs in trauma, it is usually a late manifestation. Neurogenic shock occurs when an injury affects the sympathetic pathway resulting in loss of sympathetic tone to the vessels and failure to produce a tachycardia from this sympathetic pathway. Therefore, this is manifested by hypotension with bradycardia and warm extremities, which are in direct contrast to the patient in hemorrhagic shock.

SLIDES 32, 33

The initial step in managing shock in the injured patient is to **recognize its presence**. No laboratory test can definitively diagnose shock. The initial diagnosis is based on clinical appreciation of the presence of **inadequate organ perfusion and tissue oxygenation** instead of the presence of hypotension. Although the patient may initially present with hypotension, the definition of shock as an abnormality of the circulatory system that results in inadequate organ perfusion and tissue oxygenation becomes an operative tool for diagnosis and treatment. (See Appendix 1, Glossary of Frequently Confused Terms.) The severity of signs and symptoms of shock closely parallels the degree of hemorrhage. (See Table 1, Estimated Fluid and Blood Losses Based on Patient's Initial Presentation.)

1. Blood volume and cardiac output

Hypotension following injury must be considered to be hypovolemic in origin until proved otherwise. Rapid and accurate assessment of the injured patient's hemodynamic status is therefore essential. The elements of clinical observation that yield key information within seconds are level of consciousness, skin color, and pulse. In assessing organ perfusion, signs accompanying decreased blood flow resulting from a decrease in cardiac output should be sought, for example, tachycardia, cool extremities from vasoconstriction, narrowed pulse pressure, and in the later phases, a fall in mean arterial blood pressure. Ideally, the diagnosis of shock should be made prior to the development of obvious hypotension.

a. Level of consciousness

When circulating blood volume is reduced, cerebral perfusion may be critically impaired, resulting in altered levels of consciousness. However, a conscious patient also may have lost a significant amount of blood.

b. Skin color and capillary refill

Skin color can be helpful in evaluating the hypovolemic injured patient. A patient with normal capillary refill (<2 seconds) and pink skin, especially in the face and extremities, is rarely critically hypovolemic after injury. Conversely, the ashen, gray skin of the face and the white skin of the exsanguinated extremities are ominous signs of hypovolemia.

c. **Pulse**

An easily accessible central pulse (femoral or carotid, or in an infant, brachial), should be assessed bilaterally for quality, rate, and regularity. Full, slow, and regular peripheral pulses are **usually** signs of relative normovolemia in a patient who has not been taking beta-adrenergic blocking medications. A rapid, thready pulse is usually a sign of hypovolemia, but may have other causes as well. A normal pulse rate does not assure that the patient is normovolemic. An irregular pulse usually is a warning of potential cardiac dysfunction. Absent central pulses, not attributable to local factors, signify the need for immediate resuscitative action to control hemorrhage and restore depleted blood volume and effective cardiac output if death is to be avoided.

2. Special considerations

SLIDE 34

Children, the elderly, athletes, pregnant women, and others with chronic medical conditions do not respond to volume loss in similar or even in a "normal" manner.

Thus, anticipation and an attitude of skepticism regarding the patient's "normal" hemodynamic status are appropriate.

a. Children usually have abundant physiologic reserve and often demonstrate few signs of hypovolemia even after severe volume depletion. When deterioration does occur, it is precipitous and catastrophic.

b. The elderly, at the other extreme, have a limited ability to increase their heart rate in response to blood loss, obscuring one of the earliest signs of volume depletion, tachycardia. Blood pressure has little correlation with cardiac output in the older patient group.

c. The well-trained athlete also has vigorous compensatory mechanisms, is normally relatively bradycardic, and does not demonstrate the usual level of tachycardia with blood loss.

d. Pregnant women also have an altered response to volume loss. Due to the physiologic hypervolemia of pregnancy and catecholamine-stimulated vasoconstriction in the placental circulation, significant volume loss may occur before signs of hypovolemia become apparent.

e. It also is common that the "AMPLE" history, described subsequently in this chapter, is not possible to obtain, and the health care team is not aware of the patient's use of medications for chronic conditions.

3. Bleeding

SLIDES 35, 36, 37

Bleeding should be considered external or internal. **External hemorrhage is identified by physical examination and promptly controlled by direct pressure in the primary survey.** As indicated previously, an internal source of hemorrhage may be identified by a combination of history, physical examination, and simple investigations such as chest X ray, X ray of the pelvis, FAST, and CT in the patient who is not hemodynamically compromised.

Large-bore IV access is established for fluid resuscitation beginning with Ringer's lactate or normal saline followed by blood if necessary. In penetrating torso trauma without head injury, the main goal is to stop the hemorrhage, which may require surgical intervention. The hemodynamic endpoints of fluid resuscitation prior to surgery in these cases may involve maintaining borderline hypotension to decrease possible blood loss prior to surgery.

Table 1 Estimated Fluid and Blood Losses[1] Based on Patient's Initial Presentation				
	Class I	**Class II**	**Class III**	**Class IV**
Blood loss (mL)	Up to 750	750–1500	1500–2000	>2000
Blood loss (% blood volume)	Up to 15%	15%–30%	30%–40%	>40%
Heart rate	<100	>100	>120	>140
Blood pressure	Normal	Normal	Decreased	Decreased
Pulse pressure (mm Hg)	Normal	Decreased	Decreased	Decreased
Respiratory rate	14–20	20–30	30–40	>35
Urine output (mL/hr)	>30	20–30	5–15	Negligible
CNS mental status	Slightly anxious	Mildly anxious	Anxious, confused	Confused, lethargic
Fluid replacement (3:1 rule)	Crystalloid	Crystalloid	Crystalloid and blood	Crystalloid and blood

[1]*For a 70-kg man.*

Stopping the hemorrhage takes priority over fluid administration, and this may require operative intervention. The guidelines in Table 1 are based on the "3-for-1" rule. This rule derives from the empiric observation that most patients in hemorrhagic shock require as much as 300 mL of electrolyte solution for each 100 mL of blood loss. Applied blindly, these guidelines can result in excessive or inadequate fluid administration. For example, a patient with a crush injury to the extremity may have hypotension out of proportion to his or her blood loss and require fluids in excess of the 3:1 guidelines. In contrast, a patient whose continuing blood loss is being replaced by blood transfusion requires less than 3:1. The use of bolus therapy with careful monitoring of the patient's response can moderate these extremes.

Rapid, external blood loss is managed by direct manual pressure on the wound. Pneumatic splinting devices also may help control hemorrhage. These devices should be transparent to allow monitoring of underlying bleeding. Tourniquets should **not** be used because they crush tissues and cause distal ischemia, except in unusual circumstances such as a traumatic amputation of an extremity. The use of hemostats is time-consuming and surrounding structures, such as nerves and veins, can be injured. Hemorrhage into the thoracic or abdominal cavities, soft tissues surrounding a major long bone fracture, the retroperitoneal space from a pelvic fracture, or as a result of a penetrating torso injury are the major sources of occult blood loss.

4. Life-threatening chest injuries causing shock

A patient with injuries above the diaphragm may demonstrate evidence of inadequate organ perfusion due to poor cardiac performance from blunt or penetrating myocardial injury, cardiac tamponade, tension pneumothorax that produces inadequate venous return, or massive bleeding into the chest cavity. (See Appendix 1, Glossary of Frequently Confused Terms.)

a. Tension pneumothorax

Tension pneumothorax is a true surgical emergency that requires immediate diagnosis and treatment. Tension pneumothorax develops when air enters the pleural space but a flap-valve mechanism prevents its escape. Intrapleural pressure rises, causing total lung collapse and a shift of the mediastinum to the opposite side with subsequent impairment of venous return and fall in cardiac output. Tension pneumothorax initially causes chest pain and acute respiratory distress. It also may cause hypotension as compression of the superior and/or inferior vena cava, at the upper and lower thoracic inlets, decreases venous return. Tension pneumothorax is a clinical diagnosis, and treatment should not be delayed by waiting for radiologic confirmation. It requires immediate needle decompression, followed by tube thoracostomy.

b. Massive hemothorax

Massive hemothorax may acutely impair ventilation when more than 1500 mL of blood rapidly accumulates in the chest cavity. However, it more dramatically presents as hypotension and shock. Massive hemothorax is initially managed by the simultaneous restoration of blood volume and decompression of the chest cavity by means of tube thoracostomy. If 1500 mL of blood is immediately evacuated, it is highly likely that the patient will require an early thoracotomy for control of hemorrhage.

c. Cardiac tamponade

Cardiac tamponade may be caused by bleeding into the pericardium from the heart, great vessels, or pericardial vessels. Only a relatively small amount of blood is required to restrict cardiac activity and interfere with cardiac filling. When the diagnosis of cardiac tamponade is first considered, intravenous fluid should be infused as fast as possible since increasing the preload to the heart will temporarily raise the patient's blood pressure. Prompt evacuation of pericardial blood (pericardiocentesis or preferably pericardiotomy if expertise is immediately available) is indicated for patients who do not respond to the usual measures of resuscitation for hemorrhagic shock and who have the potential for cardiac tamponade. Evacuating the pericardial sac should not be delayed for any diagnostic adjunct other than FAST, if immediately available, for assessing the pericardial sac for the presence of fluid. Removal of small amounts of blood or fluid, often as little as 15 to 20 mL, may result in immediate hemodynamic improvement if cardiac tamponade exists. However, this procedure must be followed by direct operative repair of the bleeding source.

D. Disability (Neurologic Status)

After circulatory assessment and management, a rapid neurologic evaluation is performed. This neurologic evaluation establishes the patient's level of consciousness as well as pupillary size and reaction.

The Glasgow Coma Scale (GCS) Score provides a quick measure of the level of consciousness. Eye opening is scored from 4 (spontaneous) to 1 (none); best motor response is scored from 6 (obeys commands) to 1 (none); verbal response is scored from 5 (oriented) to 1 (none). The GCS Score is the sum of these three, with the best possible score being 15 and the worst possible score being 3. The score is modified for pediatric patients. (See Appendix 3, Revised and Pediatric Trauma Scores.)

A decrease in the level of consciousness may indicate decreased cerebral oxygenation and/or perfusion (secondary brain injury), or it may be due to direct brain injury (primary brain injury). An altered level of consciousness indicates the need for immediate reevaluation of the patient's oxygenation, ventilation, and perfusion status. Prevention of secondary brain injury by maintenance of oxygenation, ventilation, and perfusion is the main goal of initial resuscitation of the brain-injured patient. Alcohol and/or other drugs also may alter the patient's level of consciousness. However, if hypoxia and hypovolemia are excluded, changes in the level of consciousness should be considered to be of traumatic central nervous system origin until proven otherwise. Early CT scan and neurosurgical consultation are absolutely essential in the management of the brain-injured patient.

A unilaterally dilated pupil is an ominous sign that indicates the presence of a mass lesion, usually an expanding intracranial hematoma. Failure to recognize and manage an intracranial hemorrhage can lead to transtentorial herniation and death. As intracranial volume increases due to a mass or hemorrhage from trauma, there is a compensatory fluid volume decrease in the cerebrospinal fluid and brain vessels, which tends to maintain the intracranial pressure at a lower level until a critical point is reached (Monroe-Kellie Doctrine). Once this critical point is reached, there is no further room for decreasing the volume in the brain and a rapid, massive increase in intracranial pressure leads to cerebral ischemia, uncal herniation, and death. The mass must be removed prior to this critical point if treatment, including surgical intervention, is to be effective.

In the normal brain cerebral perfusion is maintained over a wide range of blood-pressures (cerebral blood flow autoregulation) from 50–160 mm Hg. This response is disrupted in brain injury. Cerebral blood flow is also altered by the level of arterial PCO_2, hyperventilation, and hypocapnea being associated with decreased cerebral perfusion. Decreasing arterial PCO_2 for brief periods can therefore result in decreased intracranial pressure, but prolonged hypocapnea can result in cerebral ischemia.

As intracranial pressure rises, there is a compensatory increase in mean arterial pressure (Cushing's response) to maintain cerebral perfusion. Systemic hypertension should therefore not be treated in the head injured patient with increased intracranial pressure.

Despite proper attention to all aspects of managing the patient with a closed head injury, neurologic deterioration can occur, often rapidly. The lucid interval commonly associated with acute epidural hematoma is an example of a situation where the patient will "talk and die." Frequent neurologic **reevaluation** can prevent this problem by allowing early detection of changes. It may be necessary to return to the primary survey and to confirm that the patient has a secure airway, adequate ventilation and oxygenation, and adequate cerebral perfusion. Emergent consultation with the neurosurgeon also is necessary to guide additional management efforts.

SLIDE 39

SLIDE 40

SLIDE 41

SLIDES 42, 43

E. Exposure/Environmental Control

The patient should be completely undressed, usually by cutting off the garments to facilitate thorough examination and assessment. Sporting gear (for example, football helmets and shoulder pads) also should be removed at this time while observing appropriate spine precautions. After the patient's clothing is removed and assessment is completed, it is imperative to cover the patient with warm blankets or an external warming device to prevent hypothermia in the emergency department. Intravenous fluids should be warmed before infusion, and a warm environment should be maintained. **It is the patient's body temperature which is most important, not the comfort of the health care providers.**

Injured patients may arrive in the emergency department hypothermic, and some of those who require massive transfusions and crystalloid resuscitation become hypothermic despite aggressive efforts to maintain body temperature. **The problem is best minimized by early control of hemorrhage. This may require operative intervention or the application of an external device to reduce the pelvic volume for certain types of pelvic fractures.** Efforts to rewarm the patient and to prevent hypothermia should be considered as important as any other component of the primary survey or resuscitation phase!

Resuscitation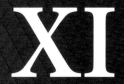

The resuscitation phase is conducted simultaneously with the primary survey. Aggressive resuscitation and the management of life-threatening injuries, as they are identified, are essential to ensure patient survival.

SLIDES 45, 46

A. Airway

The airway should be protected in all patients and secured when the potential for airway compromise exists. The **jaw thrust** or **chin lift** maneuver may suffice. A **nasopharyngeal airway** may initially establish and maintain airway patency in the conscious patient. If the patient is unconscious and has no gag reflex, an oropharyngeal airway may be helpful temporarily. **However, a definitive airway should be established if there is any doubt about the patient's ability to maintain airway integrity.**

Definitive control of the airway in patients who have compromised airways due to mechanical factors, who have ventilatory problems, or who are unconscious is achieved by endotracheal intubation, either nasally or orally (nasal intubation is contraindicated in the presence of basal skull fracture). This procedure should be accomplished with continuous protection of the cervical spine. A surgical airway (cricothyroidotomy) should be performed if oro- or nasotracheal intubation is contraindicated or cannot be accomplished. In the infant and young child, the needle cricothyroidotomy is preferred over the surgical cricothyroidotomy. This allows time (30 to 45 minutes) during which oxygenation can be maintained while arranging for a more formal surgical airway in the operating room. After 30 to 40 minutes, hypercapnea results because the narrow catheter used in this technique does not allow adequate ventilation for prolonged periods of time.

B. Breathing/Ventilation/Oxygenation

Every injured patient should receive **supplemental oxygen** to achieve optimal oxygenation. If not intubated and if the patient is breathing spontaneously, the patient should have oxygen administered by a nonrebreathing mask to achieve optimal oxygenation. If intubated, the patient should have oxygen delivered by, and ventilations assisted with, a bag-valve reservoir device. This process should be followed by mechanical ventilation after excluding a pneumothorax, which will require a tube thoracostomy. The use of the pulse oximeter is valuable in monitoring adequate hemoglobin oxygen saturation.

Tube thoracostomy is required in the definitive control of the following, immediately life-threatening chest injuries.

1. Tension pneumothorax, after needle decompression
2. Open pneumothorax, after placement of an occlusive dressing over the wound
3. Massive hemothorax with simultaneous restoration of blood volume

C. Circulation

The first, most critical step in hemorrhagic shock management is to identify and stop the bleeding. **Control bleeding by direct pressure or operative intervention**. With few exceptions, patients who are hypotensive from hemorrhage on admission require urgent surgical management.

The second vitally important step in shock management, **after hemorrhage is controlled**, is to restore circulating blood volume. A minimum of **two large-caliber intravenous catheters** (IVs) should be established. The maximum rate of fluid administration is determined by the internal diameter of the catheter and inversely by its length, not by the size of the vein in which the catheter is placed. Therefore, large-caliber, short catheters are preferred. Establishment of upper extremity peripheral intravenous access is preferred. Other peripheral lines, cutdowns, and central venous lines should be utilized as necessary in accordance with the skill level of the doctor caring for the patient. When establishing the intravenous lines, blood should be drawn for type and crossmatch and for baseline hematology studies, including a pregnancy test for all females of childbearing age.

Intravenous fluid therapy with a balanced salt solution should be initiated. Ringer's lactate solution or normal saline is the initial crystalloid solution and should be administered rapidly. Such bolus intravenous therapy may require the administration of 2 to 3 liters of solution within minutes to achieve an appropriate patient response in the adult patient. All intravenous solutions should be **warmed** either by storage in a warm environment (37° to 40°C or 98.6° to 104°F) or by fluid warming devices.

The shock state associated with trauma is most often hypovolemic in origin. Patients with minimal blood loss (less than 20% blood loss) respond rapidly to bolus intravenous therapy. However, if the patient responds only transiently to fluid replacement or remains unresponsive to bolus intravenous therapy, **type-specific blood** may be administered as necessary. If type-specific blood is not available, **low titer type O or O-negative blood** is considered as a substitute. For life-threatening blood loss, the use of unmatched, type-specific blood is preferred over type O blood unless multiple, unidentified casualties are being treated simultaneously or the patient's hypotensive state does not permit the time necessary for typing. Hypovolemic shock should not be treated by vasopressors, steroids, or sodium bicarbonate, **or** continued crystalloid/blood infusion. If blood loss continues this should be controlled by **operative intervention**. The process of operative resuscitation provides the surgeon the opportunity to stop the bleeding **in addition to** the maintaining and restoring intravascular volume. If shock persists despite seemingly adequate volume resuscitation, consider other causes of shock, for example, tension pneumothorax, cardiac tamponade, and blunt cardiac injury.

Hypothermia may be present when the patient arrives, or it may develop quickly in the emergency department in the uncovered patient and by rapid administration of room temperature fluids or refrigerated blood. Hypothermia is a potentially lethal complication in the injured patient, and aggressive measures should be taken to prevent the loss of body heat and to restore body temperature to normal. **The temperature of the resuscitation area should be increased to minimize the loss of body heat**. The use of a high-flow fluid warmer or microwave oven to heat crystalloid fluids to 39°C (102.2°F) is recommended. Blood products should not be warmed in a microwave oven.

Adjuncts to Primary Survey and Resuscitation

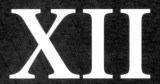

A. Urinary and Gastric Catheters

The placement of urinary and gastric catheters should be considered as part of the resuscitation phase.

1. Urinary catheters

Urinary output is a sensitive indicator of the volume status of the patient and reflects renal perfusion. Monitoring of urinary output is best accomplished by the insertion of an indwelling bladder catheter. Transurethral bladder catheterization is contraindicated in patients in whom urethral injury is suspected. Urethral injury should be suspected if there is (1) blood at the penile meatus, (2) perineal ecchymosis, (3) scrotal hematoma, (4) a high-riding or nonpalpable prostate, or (5) a pelvic fracture. Therefore, the urinary catheter should not be inserted before an examination of the rectum and genitalia if the mechanism of injury suggests the possibility of urethral injury. If urethral injury is suspected, urethral integrity should be confirmed by a retrograde urethrogram before the catheter is inserted.

SLIDE 47

A urine specimen should be submitted for routine laboratory analysis whenever a urinary catheter is inserted.

2. Gastric catheters

A gastric tube is indicated to reduce stomach distention and decrease the risk of aspiration. Decompression of the stomach reduces the risk of aspiration, **but does not prevent it entirely.** Thick or semisolid gastric contents will not return through the tube, and actual passage of the tube may induce vomiting. For the tube to be effective, it must be positioned properly, attached to appropriate suction, and be functioning. Blood in the gastric aspirate may represent oropharyngeal (swallowed) blood, traumatic insertion, or actual injury to the upper digestive tract. If a cribriform plate fracture, basilar skull fracture, or maxillofacial trauma is suspected or present, the gastric tube should be inserted orally to prevent intracranial passage. In this situation, any nasopharyngeal instrumentation is potentially dangerous.

SLIDE 48

SLIDE 49

B. Monitoring

Adequate resuscitation is best assessed by improvement in physiologic parameters—for example, pulse rate, blood pressure, pulse pressure, ventilatory rate, arterial blood gas analysis, body temperature, and urinary output—rather than the qualitative assessment done in the primary survey. **Actual values for these parameters should be obtained as soon as practical after completing the primary survey. Periodic reevaluation is important.**

1. **Ventilatory rate and arterial blood gases** should be used to monitor the adequacy of the patient's airway and breathing. Endotracheal tubes can be dislodged whenever the patient is moved. A colorimetric carbon dioxide detector should be readily available in the emergency department. This device can rapidly detect the presence of carbon dioxide in exhaled gas, provided the patient is in a perfusing cardiac rhythm. It is useful in confirming that the endotracheal tube is located somewhere in the airway of the ventilated patient and not in the esophagus. It does not confirm proper placement of the tube in the airway. Auscultation of the chest and epigastrium, as well as a chest x-ray, are also important for determining tube position.

2. **Pulse oximetry** is a valuable adjunct for monitoring injured patients. The pulse oximeter measures the oxygen saturation of hemoglobin colorimetrically, but does **not** measure ventilation or the partial pressure of oxygen. A small sensor is placed on the finger, toe, earlobe, or some other convenient area of the skin. Most devices display pulse rate and oxygen saturation continuously.

3. **Blood pressure** should be measured serially and recorded. Keep in mind that it may be a poor measure of actual tissue perfusion.

4. **Electrocardiographic (ECG) monitoring** of all trauma patients is required. Dysrhythmias, including unexplained tachycardia, atrial fibrillation, premature ventricular contractions, and pulseless electrical activity (PEA, formerly termed electromechanical dissociation), may indicate cardiac tamponade, tension pneumothorax, and/or profound hypovolemia. When bradycardia, aberrant conduction, and premature beats are present, hypoxia and hypoperfusion

C. X rays and Diagnostic Studies

X rays should be used judiciously and should not delay patient resuscitation. The anteroposterior (AP) chest film and an AP pelvis film may provide information that can guide resuscitation efforts of the patient with blunt trauma. Chest films may demonstrate potentially life-threatening injuries requiring treatment, and pelvic films may demonstrate fractures of the pelvis which indicate the need for early blood transfusion and the possibility of urethral or bladder injury. These films can be taken in the resuscitation area, usually with a portable X ray unit, but should not interrupt the resuscitation process.

A lateral cervical spine X ray or CT scan should be obtained with a portable X ray unit during the secondary survey on any patient who may have a cervical spine injury. A lateral cervical spine X ray that demonstrates an injury is an important finding, while a negative or inadequate film does not exclude cervical spine injury. During the secondary survey, complete cervical and thoracolumbar spine films also may be obtained if the patient's care is not compromised, and if the mechanism of injury or physical examination suggests the possibility of spinal injury. Spinal cord protection, by maintaining bimanual inline stabilization, followed by application of appropriate spinal immobilization devices (eg, semirigid cervical extrication collar, long spine board, and commercial head immobilizer), should be the goal during the primary survey rather than obtaining X rays. Patients with no history of loss of consciousness who are alert and have no symptoms or signs in the neck or no neurologic deficit, may not require c-spine X rays before removing the cervical extrication collar. **Essential** diagnostic X rays should **not** be avoided in the pregnant patient.

Diagnostic peritoneal lavage (DPL) and focused assessment sonography in trauma (FAST) are useful tools for the quick detection of occult intraabdominal bleeding. Their use depends on the skill and experience level of the doctor. Early identification of the source of occult intraabdominal blood loss may indicate the need for operative control of hemorrhage. FAST is more rapid and less invasive, but operator dependent. A CT scan of the abdomen is more specific than FAST, but because it requires moving the patient to the CT scan suite, it is only appropriate when the patient's hemodynamics have been normalized.

Notes:

Consider Need for Patient Transfer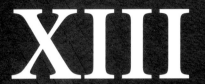

During the primary survey and resuscitation phase, the evaluating doctor frequently has enough information to indicate the need for transfer of the patient to another facility. This transfer process may be initiated immediately by administrative personnel at the direction of the examining doctor while additional evaluation and resuscitative measures are being performed. Transfer should be initiated when the treatment needs of the patient exceed the capabilities of the initial facility. The patient should be transferred to the closest appropriate facility—for example, one capable of satisfactorily meeting the patient's treatment needs, ideally a trauma center. Once the decision to transfer the patient has been made, referring doctor to receiving doctor communication is essential. Unnecessary diagnostic studies such as X rays and CT scans should not be conducted prior to transfer, as they may delay the transfer process. **Remember**, life-saving measures are initiated when a problem is identified, rather than after the primary survey is completed.

Notes:

Secondary Survey

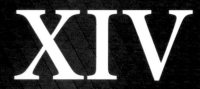

The secondary survey does not begin until the primary survey (ABCDEs) is completed, resuscitative efforts are well established, and the patient is demonstrating normalization of vital functions.

SLIDE 50

The secondary survey is a **head-to-toe evaluation** of the trauma patient, that is, a complete history and physical examination, including a **reassessment** of all vital signs. Each region of the body is completely examined. The potential for missing an injury or failing to appreciate the significance of an injury is great, especially in the unresponsive or unstable patient.

SLIDE 51

In this survey a complete neurologic examination is performed, including a GCS Score determination, if not done during the primary survey. During this evaluation, indicated X rays (for example, X rays pertinent to the sites of suspected injury) are obtained. Such examinations can be interspersed into the secondary survey at appropriate times.

Special procedures—for example, specific radiologic evaluations and laboratory studies—also are performed during this time. Complete evaluation of the patient requires repeated physical examination. The secondary assessment might well be summarized as "tubes and fingers in every orifice."

A. History

Every complete medical assessment should include a history of the mechanism of injury. Many times such a history cannot be obtained from the patient. Prehospital personnel and family must be consulted to obtain information that may enhance an understanding of the patient's physiologic state. The AMPLE history is a useful mnemonic for this purpose.

(A) **A**llergies

(M) **M**edications currently used

(P) **P**ast illnesses/Pregnancy

(L) **L**ast meal

(E) **E**vents/**E**nvironment related to the injury

SLIDE 52

The patient's condition is greatly influenced by the mechanism of injury. Prehospital personnel can provide valuable information on such mechanisms and should report pertinent data to the examining doctor. Some injuries can be predicted based on the direction and amount of energy force. (See Appendix 4, Mechanisms of Automotive Injury and Related, Suspected Injury Patterns.) Injury usually is classified into two broad categories, blunt and penetrating.

SLIDE 53

1. Blunt trauma

Blunt trauma results from automobile collisions, falls, and other transportation-, recreation-, and occupation-related injuries. Important information to obtain about automobile collisions includes seat belt usage, airbag deployment, steering wheel deformation, direction of impact, damage to the automobile in terms of major deformation or intrusion into the passenger compartment, and ejection of the passenger from the vehicle. Ejection from the vehicle greatly increases the chance of major injury.

Injury patterns may often be predicted by the mechanism of injury. Such injury patterns also are influenced by age groups and activities. (See Appendix 4, Mechanisms of Automotive Injury and Related, Suspected Injury Patterns.)

2. Penetrating trauma

Injuries from penetrating trauma (firearms, stabbings, and impaling objects) are seen around the world. Factors determining the type and extent of injury and subsequent management include the region of the body injured, the organs in proximity to the path of the penetrating object, and the velocity of the missile. Therefore, the velocity, caliber, presumed path of the bullet, and the distance from weapon to wounded may provide important clues to the extent of injury.

3. Injuries due to burns and cold

SLIDES 54, 55, 56

Burns are another significant type of trauma that may occur alone or may be coupled with blunt and penetrating trauma resulting from a burning automobile, explosion, falling debris, the patient's attempt to escape the fire, or an assault with a firearm or knife. Inhalation injury and carbon monoxide poisoning often complicate burn injury. Such complications require early intubation, mechanical ventilation, and the administration of 100 percent oxygen. Therefore, it is important to know the circumstances of the burn injury. Specifically, knowledge of the environment in which the burn injury occurred (open or closed space), substances consumed by the flames (plastics, chemicals, and so on), and possible associated injuries sustained is critical in the treatment of the patient.

Fluid resuscitation of the burn patient requires an estimate of the area of the burn (second degree or greater), the weight of the patient, and the time of the burn injury. The rule of nines is a practical guide for estimating the body surface area (BSA) of the burn. The adult body is divided into anatomic regions representing 9 percent or multiples of 9 percent In children, the head represents a larger percentage and the lower limbs a lower percentage of the surface area when compared to the adult. The palmar surface of the patient's hand represents 1percent of BSA. With these parameters, the estimated 24-hour volume of crystalloid (Ringer's lactate) infusion is 2 to 4 mL/kg/% BSA of burn. One half of this volume is administered in the first eight hours after the injury and the second half in the next 16 hours. In infants and young children, maintenance fluid also must be administered. This estimated volume requirement is used only as a guide, the actual volume administered being determined by the adequacy of perfusion as indicated by hemodynamic parameters and urinary output.

Patients sustaining body surface chemical burns require removal of dry chemicals and/or profuse irrigation of the affected area.

Pediatric

Adult

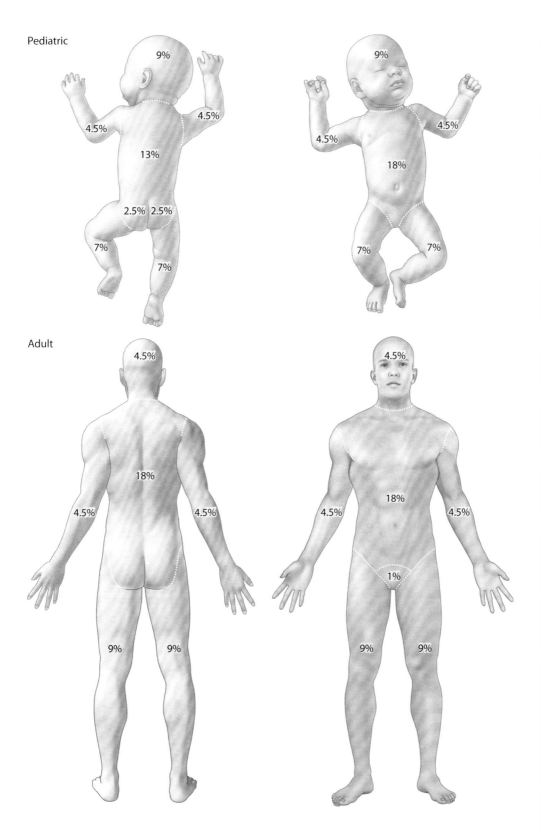

*Advanced Trauma Life Support for Doctors
Student Course Manual, 8e*
**American College of Surgeons
Figure# 09.01
Dragonfly Media Group**

Figure 6 Rule of Nines.
This practical guide is used to evaluate the severity of
burns and determine fluid management. The adult body
is generally divided into surface areas of 9% each and/or
fractions or multiples of 9%.

Acute or chronic hypothermia without adequate protection against heat loss produces either local or generalized cold injuries. Significant heat loss may occur at moderate temperatures (15° to 20°C or 59° to 68°F) if wet clothes, decreased activity, or vasodilatation caused by alcohol or drugs compromises the patient's ability to conserve heat. Such historical information can be obtained from prehospital personnel.

The most significant local cold injury is frostbite because of its associated risk of tissue or limb loss. The most significant generalized cold injury is hypothermia (core temperature less than 35°C [95°F]) because of its major systemic effects, which can be lethal. Frostbite treatment requires removal from the cold environment, rapid rewarming with moist heat (water tank at 40°C [104°F]), and waiting for demarcation before debridement. Hypothermia treatment also requires removal from the cold environment, the use of warming devices that may be passive or active, while monitoring temperature, hemodynamics, and coagulation parameters. Unless the hypothermic patient has a previous cardiovascular or hypoxic insult leading to the hypothermia and loss of vital signs, the patient cannot be pronounced dead until warming techniques are instituted and the patient's core temperature is reversed, because with rewarming the lack of vital signs also can be reversed.

4. Hazardous environment

History of exposure to chemicals, toxins, and radiation is important to obtain for two reasons. First, these agents can produce a variety of pulmonary, cardiac, or internal organ dysfunction in the injured patient. Second, these same agents also present a hazard to health care providers. Frequently, the doctor's only means of preparation is to understand the general principles of management of such conditions and establish immediate contact with the regional Poison Control Center.

B. Physical Examination

1. Head

SLIDE 57

The secondary survey begins with evaluating the head and identifying all related and significant injuries. The entire scalp and head should be examined for lacerations, contusions, and evidence of fractures. Because edema around the eyes may later preclude an in-depth examination, the eyes should be reevaluated for:

a. Visual acuity

b. Pupillary size

c. Hemorrhages of the conjunctiva and fundi

d. Penetrating injury

e. Contact lenses (remove before edema occurs)

f. Dislocation of the lens

g. Ocular entrapment

A quick visual acuity examination of both eyes can be performed by having the patient read printed material, for example, a hand-held Snelling Chart or words on an intravenous container or a 4 x 4 dressing package. Ocular mobility should be evaluated to exclude entrapment of extraocular muscles due to orbital fractures. These procedures frequently identify optic injuries not otherwise apparent.

Facial edema in patients with massive facial injury or patients in coma can preclude a complete eye examination. Such difficulties should not deter the doctor from performing those components of the ocular examination that are possible.

2. Maxillofacial

SLIDE 58

Maxillofacial trauma not associated with airway obstruction or major bleeding should be treated only after the patient is stabilized completely and life-threatening injuries have been managed. Definitive management may be safely delayed without compromising care at the discretion of appropriate specialists.

Patients with fractures of the midface may have a fracture of the cribriform plate. For these patients, gastric intubation should be performed via the oral route.

Some maxillofacial fractures—for example, nasal fracture, nondisplaced zygomatic fractures, and orbital rim fractures—may be difficult to identify early in the evaluation process. Therefore, frequent reassessment is crucial.

3. Cervical spine and neck

SLIDE 59

Patients with maxillofacial or head trauma should be presumed to have an unstable cervical spine injury (fracture and/or ligamentous injury), and the neck should be immobilized until all aspects of the cervical spine have been adequately studied, injury has been excluded, and the patient is clinically asymptomatic. The absence of neurologic deficit does not exclude injury to the cervical spine, and such injury should be presumed until a complete cervical spine radiographic series is reviewed by a doctor experienced in detecting cervical spine fractures radiographically.

Deciding that a spinal injury is absent requires negative clinical and radiologic findings in the absence of other painful injuries that may distract the patient's attention from pain of spinal origin. If the patient has no signs of spine injury clinically, is alert, and has not lost consciousness, the cervical extrication collar may be removed without imaging of the spine. When imaging is considered necessary, it should include anteroposterior (AP) and lateral views with visualization of all the cervical vertebrae to the top of T1, and an open-mouth odontoid view. AP and lateral thoracic and lumbar spine X rays also may be required. The absence of radiologic findings must be corroborated by physical findings before the spine is declared normal. If spine injury is suspected and one is unable to conduct an appropriate clinical examination to detect signs of spine injury (for example, the head-injured or unconscious patient, or a patient with an altered sensorium), the cervical extrication collar must be left in place and the patient considered as having a spine injury until proven otherwise. Imaging techniques such as CT scan, MRI, and flexion and extension views of the spine may be required later and are obtained and interpreted by personnel (for example, orthopaedic surgeon, neurosurgeon, or radiologist) experienced in these techniques.

SLIDE 60

Examination of the neck includes inspection, palpation, and auscultation. Cervical spine tenderness, subcutaneous emphysema, tracheal deviation, and laryngeal fracture may be discovered on a detailed examination. The carotid arteries should be palpated and auscultated for bruits. Evidence of blunt injury over these vessels should be noted and, if present, should arouse a high index of suspicion for carotid artery injury. Occlusion or dissection of the carotid artery may occur hours or days after the injury without antecedent signs or symptoms. Angiography or duplex ultrasonography may be required to exclude the possibility of major cervical vascular injury when the mechanism of injury suggests that possibility. Most major cervical vascular injuries are the result of penetrating injury. However, blunt force to the neck or a traction injury from a shoulder harness restraint can result in intimal disruption, dissection, and thrombosis.

Protection of a potentially unstable cervical spine is imperative for patients wearing any type of protective helmet. Extreme care must be taken when removing the helmet.

Penetrating injuries to the neck have the potential of injuring several organ systems. Wounds that extend through the platysma should not be explored manually or probed with instruments in the emergency department or by individuals in the emergency department who are not trained to deal with such injuries. The emergency department usually is not equipped to deal with problems, which may be encountered unexpectedly. These injuries require evaluation by a surgeon, either operatively or with specialized diagnostic procedures under direct supervision by the surgeon. The finding of active arterial bleeding, an expanding hematoma, arterial bruit, or airway compromise usually requires surgical operative evaluation. Unexplained or isolated paralysis of an upper extremity should raise the suspicion of a cervical nerve root injury and be accurately documented.

Blunt injury to the neck may be associated with the development of late clinical signs and symptoms, which may not be evident during the initial examination. Injury to the intima of the carotid arteries is an example.

The identification of cervical nerve root or brachial plexus injury may not be possible in the comatose patient. Consideration of the mechanism of injury may be the only clue available to the doctor.

In some patients, a decubitus ulcer may develop quickly over the sacrum or other areas from immobilization on a rigid spine board and the cervical collar. Efforts to exclude the possibility of spinal injury should be initiated as soon as practical and these devices removed. However, resuscitation and efforts to identify life-threatening or potentially life-threatening injuries should not be compromised.

4. Chest

A complete evaluation of the chest wall requires inspection and palpation of the entire chest cage, including the clavicle, ribs, and sternum. Sternal pressure may be painful if the sternum is fractured or costochondral separations exist. Contusions and hematomas of the chest wall should alert the doctor to the possibility of occult injury.

Significant chest injury may be manifested by pain, dyspnea, or hypoxia. Evaluation includes auscultation of the chest and a chest X ray. Breath sounds are auscultated high on the anterior chest wall for pneumothorax and at the posterior bases for hemothorax. Auscultatory findings may be difficult to evaluate in a noisy environment but may be extremely helpful. Distant heart sounds and narrow pulse pressure may indicate cardiac tamponade. Cardiac tamponade or tension pneumothorax may be suggested by the presence of distended neck veins, although associated hypovolemia may minimize this finding or eliminate it altogether. Decreased breath sounds, hyperresonance to percussion, and shock may be the only indications of tension pneumothorax and the need for immediate chest decompression, which should have been identified and treated during the primary survey.

Significant injury to the intrathoracic structures, especially the lungs, occurs frequently in children without evidence of thoracic skeletal trauma on physical examination. A high index of suspicion is essential.

Elderly patients may not be tolerant of even relatively minor chest injuries. Progression to acute respiratory insufficiency must be anticipated and support instituted before collapse occurs.

5. Abdomen

SLIDE 62

Abdominal injuries must be identified and treated aggressively. The specific diagnosis is not as important as the recognition that an injury exists and surgical intervention may be necessary. A normal initial examination of the abdomen does not exclude a significant intraabdominal injury. Close observation and frequent reevaluation of the abdomen, preferably by the same observer, is important in managing blunt abdominal trauma. Over time, the patient's abdominal findings may change. Early involvement by a surgeon is essential.

Patients with unexplained hypotension, neurologic injury, impaired sensorium secondary to alcohol and/or other drugs, and equivocal abdominal findings should be considered as candidates for peritoneal lavage, abdominal ultrasonography, or if hemodynamically normal, computed tomography of the abdomen with intravenous and intragastric contrast. Fractures of the pelvis or the lower rib cage also may hinder accurate diagnostic examination of the abdomen, because pain from these areas may be elicited when palpating the abdomen.

Excessive manipulation of the pelvis should be avoided. The AP pelvic X ray, performed as an adjunct to the primary survey and resuscitation, should be used as the guide for identification of pelvic fractures, which can be associated with significant blood loss.

Injury to the retroperitoneal organs may be difficult to identify, even with the use of computed tomography. Hollow viscus and pancreatic injury are classic examples.

Knowledge of injury mechanism and associated injuries that can be identified, along with a high index of suspicion, is required. Despite the doctor's appropriate diligence, some of these injuries are not diagnosed initially.

6. Perineum/rectum/vagina

SLIDE 63

The perineum should be examined for contusions, hematomas, lacerations, and urethral bleeding.

A rectal examination should have been performed before placing a urinary catheter if there is suspicion of urethral injury. Rectal examination allows assessment for the presence of blood within the bowel lumen, a high-riding prostate, the presence of pelvic fractures, the integrity of the rectal wall, and the quality of the sphincter tone.

For the female patient, a vaginal examination also is an essential part of the secondary survey. The doctor should assess for the presence of blood in the vaginal vault and vaginal lacerations. Additionally, pregnancy tests should be performed on all women of childbearing age.

Female urethral injury, while uncommon, does occur in association with pelvic fractures and straddle injuries. When present, it is difficult to detect.

7. Musculoskeletal

SLIDES 64, 65

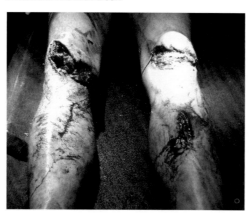

Figure 7 Example of an open fracture.

Although most musculoskeletal injuries are diagnosed and treated during the secondary survey, treatment may be required during the primary survey when life-threatening hemorrhage or limb-threatening injury results from vascular injury or ischemia from compartment syndrome. During the secondary survey, the extremities should be inspected for open wounds, contusions, or deformities. Palpation of the bones and examination for tenderness or abnormal movement aid in the identification of occult fractures. Additionally, assessment of peripheral pulses aids in the identification of vascular injuries.

Thoracic and lumbar spinal fractures, as well as neurologic injuries, must be considered based on physical findings and mechanism of injury. Other injuries may mask the physical findings of spinal injuries, which may go unsuspected unless the doctor obtains the appropriate X rays.

The doctor must remember that the musculoskeletal examination is not complete without an examination of the patient's back. Unless the patient is carefully logrolled so the patient's back can be examined, significant injuries may be missed.

Significant extremity injuries may exist without fractures being evident on examination or X rays. Ligament ruptures produce joint instability. Muscle-tendon unit injuries interfere with active motion of the affected structures. Impaired sensation and/or loss of voluntary muscle contraction strength may be due to nerve injury or to ischemia, including that due to compartment syndrome.

Fractures involving the bones of the hands, wrists, and feet are often not diagnosed in the secondary survey performed in the emergency department. It may be only after the patient has regained consciousness or other major injuries are resolved that the patient complains of pain or dysfunction in the area of an occult injury.

Compartment syndrome may be present in patients with ischemic or crush injuries to the distal lower extremities. This complication must be suspected in any patient who presents with such injuries, particularly if the patient is hypotensive or has an altered level of consciousness.

Injuries to the soft tissues around joints are frequently diagnosed after the patient begins to recover. Therefore, frequent reevaluation is essential.

SLIDE 66

Pelvic fractures can be suspected by the identification of ecchymosis over the iliac wings, pubis, labia, or scrotum. Other clues include an increase in the width of the pubic symphysis and leg length inequality. Pain on palpation of the pelvic ring is an important finding in the alert patient. Mobility of the pelvis in response to gentle anterior-to-posterior pressure with the heels of the hands on both anterior iliac spines and the symphysis pubis can suggest pelvic ring disruption in the unconscious patient.

Blood loss from pelvic fractures with increased pelvic volume can be difficult to detect and control, and fatal hemorrhage may result. A sense of urgency should accompany the management of these injuries. Fluid resuscitation and restriction of the pelvic volume by pelvic sling and external fixation devices are key elements of management. The patient's failure to respond to these measures requires consideration for angiography with the possibility of embolizing bleeding vessels.

SLIDE 67

8. Neurologic

A comprehensive neurologic examination includes not only motor and sensory evaluation of the extremities, but also reevaluation of the patient's level of consciousness and pupillary size and response. The GCS Score facilitates detection of early changes and trends in the neurologic status. (See Appendix 3, Revised and Pediatric Trauma Scores.)

SLIDE 68

Early consultation with a neurosurgeon is required for patients with neurologic injury. The patient should be monitored frequently for deterioration in the level of consciousness or changes in the neurologic examination, as these findings may reflect progression of the intracranial injury. Computed tomography (CT) of the head should be performed in any patient for whom there is suspicion of traumatic brain injury. If a patient with a head injury deteriorates neurologically, oxygenation and perfusion of the brain and the adequacy of ventilation (ABCDEs) must be reassessed, and a CT scan obtained if not already performed. Measures to reduce intracranial pressure, including intracranial surgical intervention, may be necessary. The neurosurgeon must determine whether such conditions as epidural and subdural hematomas require evacuation or depressed skull fractures need operative intervention.

Any increase in intracranial pressure can reduce cerebral perfusion pressure and lead to secondary brain injury. Secondary brain injury is caused by hypotension and hypoxia. Hypotension increases mortality. Many diagnostic and therapeutic maneuvers necessary for the evaluation and care of the brain-injured patient increase intracranial pressure. Tracheal intubation is a typical example, and in the patient with brain injury it should be performed expeditiously and as smoothly as possible. Rapid neurologic deterioration of the brain-injured patient can occur despite the application of all measures to control intracranial pressure and maintain appropriate support of the central nervous system.

Any evidence of loss of sensation, paralysis, or weakness suggests major injury to the spinal column or peripheral nervous system. X rays of the entire spinal column are indicated under such circumstances. Neurologic deficits should be documented when identified. This is especially important when transfer to another facility or doctor for specialty care is necessary. Immobilization of the entire patient, using a long spine board, a semirigid cervical collar, and/or other cervical immobilization devices, must be maintained until spinal injury can be excluded. The common mistake of immobilizing the head and freeing the torso allows the cervical spine to flex with the body as a fulcrum. Protection of the spinal cord is required at all times until a spine injury is excluded, and especially during patient transport.

SLIDES 69, 70

Notes:

Adjuncts to the Secondary Survey

XV

SLIDE 71

Specialized diagnostic tests may be performed during the secondary survey to identify specific injuries. These tests include additional X rays of the spine and extremities; computerized tomography of the head, chest, abdomen, and spine; contrast urography; angiography; transesophageal ultrasound; bronchoscopy; esophagoscopy; and other diagnostic procedures. Often these procedures require transportation of the patient to other areas of the hospital where equipment and personnel to manage life-threatening contingencies are not immediately available. Therefore, these specialized tests should not be performed until the patient's hemodynamic status has been normalized and the patient has been carefully examined. If the studies are to be performed and if there is any potential for deterioration of the patient's condition, qualified members of the trauma team must accompany the patient to the diagnostic suite.

Notes:

Reevaluation

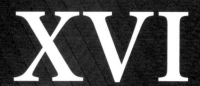

The trauma patient must be reevaluated constantly to assure that occult or other injuries (not previously identified) are not overlooked, and to discover adverse changes from previously noted findings. As initial life-threatening injuries are managed, other equally life-threatening problems and less severe injuries may become apparent. Underlying medical problems that may severely affect the ultimate prognosis of the patient may become evident. A high index of suspicion facilitates early diagnosis and management.

SLIDE 72

Continuous monitoring of vital signs and urinary output is essential. For the adult patient, maintenance of urinary output of 0.5 mL/kg/hour is desirable. In the pediatric patient over one year of age, an output of 1 mL/kg/hour should be adequate. Arterial blood gas and cardiac monitoring devices should be employed. Pulse oximetry, for critically injured patients, and end-tidal carbon dioxide monitoring, for intubated patients, should be considered.

Notes:

Pain Management

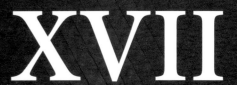

The relief of severe pain is an important part of the management of the trauma patient. Many injuries, especially musculoskeletal injuries, produce pain and anxiety in the conscious patient. Effective analgesia usually requires the use of intravenous opiates or anxiolytics. Intramuscular injections should be avoided. These agents should be administered judiciously, intravenously, and in small doses to achieve the desired level of patient comfort and relief of anxiety while avoiding respiratory depression, the masking of subtle injuries, or changes in the patient's hemodynamic status. Careful reevaluation is essential to ensure that respiratory depression does not result in impaired ventilation and oxygenation.

SLIDE 73

Notes:

Transfer to Definitive Care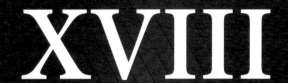

Preestablished criteria for interhospital transfer help determine the level, pace, and intensity of initial management of the multiply injured patient. These criteria take into account the patient's physiologic status, obvious anatomic injury, mechanisms of injury, concurrent diseases, and factors that may alter the patient's prognosis. Emergency department and surgical personnel should use these criteria to determine if the patient requires transfer to a trauma center or closest appropriate hospital capable of providing more specialized care. The closest appropriate hospital should be chosen based on its overall capabilities to care for the injured patient. (See Appendix 2, Prehospital Triage Decision Scheme.) Definitive care is initiated in accordance with the principles outlined herein.

SLIDE 74, 75

The transfer process should be initiated as soon as the need is recognized. Patient transfer is not delayed to obtain definitive diagnostic tests. Instead, time before transfer focuses on patient evaluation and resuscitation as well as direct doctor-to-doctor communication at the receiving hospital. Appendix 5, Guidelines for Managing the Injured Patient, serves as a checklist to guide the management of the injured patient.

Notes:

Emergency Preparedness and Disaster Management

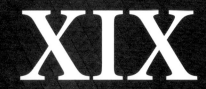

Natural- and human-caused disasters have gained much attention in recent years. Although terrorist events constitute a minority of such disasters, it is important to recognize that 93 percent to 98 percent of worldwide terrorist events in recent years have involved physical trauma, of which 75 percent are caused by blast injury. As such, the application of TEAM principles is essential in the treatment of terrorism victims, as well as those who are injured during the course of natural disasters. The following four steps constitute the fundamental elements of all disaster and emergency preparedness and response efforts.

A. Simple Disaster Plan

A basic and readily understood approach to mass casualty events is the key to effective disaster and emergency management. Plans that are too complex or cumbersome to remember or implement are destined to fail.

B. Incident Command Structure

An incident command structure (ICS) known to all personnel within a health care facility is vital to operational success during disasters, whether internal or external.

An ICS such as the Hospital Emergency Incident Command System developed under the auspices of the California EMS Authority (*http://www.emsa.cahwnet.gov*) establishes clear lines of responsibility and authority for all hospital personnel, thereby maximizing collaboration and minimizing conflicts during the typically chaotic first minutes and hours of the disaster or emergency response.

C. Disaster Triage Scheme

Whether the disaster is a multiple-casualty incident that strains the resources of the institution or a mass-casualty event that overwhelms them, a method for rapid identification of victims requiring priority treatment is essential. Most triage schemes utilize color-coded tags to indicate acuity (red = critical, yellow = urgent, green = delayed, and black = expectant). The goal in multiple-casualty incidents is to treat the sickest patients first, while in mass-casualty events, it is to save the greatest number of lives.

D. Traffic Control System

Controlling the flow of information, equipment, and personnel (providers, patients, the public, the press, and the like.) is of paramount importance in the disaster response, and these are the issues most often cited in after-action reports as causes of mismanagement. Redundant communications systems, reliable supply chains, and redoubtable security measures are all critical components of an effective disaster response. These assets must be tested on a regular basis through disaster drills that realistically represent the disaster scenarios most likely to be encountered by a particular facility.

Notes:

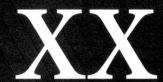

SLIDES 78, 79

The first edition of the TEAM Program Book appeared in 2000 and the second in 2005. Since that time, many dramatic and significant changes have taken place in the care of the injured patient. Further refinements in the approach to the early care of the multiply injured patient have continued to occur since that time and are reflected in this third edition.

In the rush of activity that occurs every day at every trauma center, it is easy to forget that most injuries that we see are actually preventable. In fact, the majority of deaths due to trauma occur prior to arrival at the hospital; thus, these deaths can only be impacted by prevention. Trauma care providers are, in many ways, essential to designing effective injury prevention efforts. Understanding the causes of injury and identifying the interventions that can prevent them is one of our most important contributions to our communities.

There are three categories of injury prevention. Primary prevention aims to prevent the injury before it happens. Examples of primary prevention efforts include graduated licensing laws for adolescent drivers and drunk-driving prevention programs. Secondary prevention focuses on reducing the severity of injury once it occurs. Airbags, passenger restraints, and automobile construction to provide crumple zones are included here. Tertiary prevention efforts focus on improving outcomes following injury. Creating trauma systems and assuring that patients with life-threatening injuries are transported from the scene to a trauma center are part of tertiary prevention.

In order to be effective in primary injury prevention, we need to understand how our community leadership solves problems. We have a natural role in that leadership because when we speak, our community members listen. They understand and appreciate the important role we play in **caring** for the injured. However, an organized approach aimed at **preventing** injuries requires involvement of the entire community. The following five steps serve as a quick guide on how to get started.

First, review the causes of injury and traumatic death in your community and choose a target for prevention. What you see in your trauma center is not necessarily an accurate reflection of the most important opportunities to intervene to prevent injury. For instance, there may be a neighborhood in your community with a large number of elderly residents. Although you may notice that your trauma center treats a number of elderly pedestrians struck by automobiles, unless you analyze data from the police and prehospital personnel, you will miss the opportunity to identify particularly dangerous intersections where there is a high incidence of these events. Information from community sources can really help us identify important prevention opportunities.

Second, do a good literature search to **identify proven and promising programs** that other communities have developed. You don't have time to create a new program. There is a wealth of information around the country on what works, what might work, and equally importantly, what doesn't work. For example, focusing on the elderly pedestrian, you and your community partners may find that traffic "calming" efforts that slow cars down or retiming crossing lights would be extremely effective in your area.

Third, make a plan to **draw together the agencies and organizations in your community who would make good partners in your prevention effort**. Create a collaborative partnership where each member brings his strengths to the effort. In the case of the pedestrian problem, this partnership would include the traffic division of the local police department, the local council on aging, and, perhaps, the local AARP chapter. Bringing these groups together seems daunting, but often you will find that various groups are already working on some phase of the problem. Because these efforts are fragmented and uncoordinated, no progress is being made.

Fourth, implement the program but monitor it closely and to be prepared to supply support at key steps. This step may include spending some time on the scene where prevention efforts area actually occurring. Spending time in the community is a clear sign of your interest, and you will always be welcomed as long as you pursue a strategy of collaboration. Spending an hour or two with local police at a busy intersection evaluating the effect of retiming the crossing lights for the elderly will show them that you value their efforts and will be remembered by everyone in the community.

Fifth, evaluate the results of you efforts and help revise the intervention to improve results. In our traffic prevention example, this step would include not only keeping track of the number of elderly people struck by cars but also looking at mean driving speeds in the area, number of red light running events, and other indicators that your police department's traffic division uses.

Preventing injuries should be part of **every physician's** practice, not just those who focus on their treatment. Injury prevention education for parents begins in the pediatrician's office. Every obstetrician is responsible for counseling pregnant patients on avoiding risk-taking behavior such as using drugs, drinking alcohol, or driving without being properly restrained. Medical physicians can be trained to recognize suicidal tendencies and to provide interventions for risky drinkers. Those who focus on the geriatric population have the means to prevent falls in the elderly by scrutinizing all medications. Emergency personnel may prevent fatal injuries by detecting domestic violence before it escalates. The epidemic of injury that claims the lives of so many young people can be prevented, but it will take a coordinated effort from committed physicians and community partners.

The steps in trauma prevention strategies are described in the ABCDE of trauma prevention as follows:

A **A**nalyze injury data through local injury surveillance.

B **B**uild a local coalition.

C **C**ommunicate the problem and raise local awareness that injuries are a preventable public health problem.

D **D**evelop interventions and injury prevention activities to create safer environments and activities.

E **E**valuate the interventions with ongoing surveillance.

However, for those unfortunate individuals whose injuries were not prevented, the principles presented in the TEAM Program serve as the foundation upon which effective trauma care has been established.

Summary

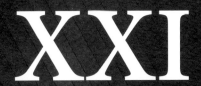

SLIDES 81, 82

The TEAM Program for medical students and multidisciplinary team members presents an ABCDE approach to trauma care. It introduces one, safe way to care for the trauma patient and emphasizes the principles of "do no further harm" and "treat the greatest threat to life first."

The injured patient must be evaluated rapidly and thoroughly. The doctor must develop treatment priorities for the overall management of the patient, so no steps in the process are omitted. An adequate patient history and accounting of the incident are important in evaluating and managing the trauma patient.

Evaluation and care are divided into the following phases for the purposes of discussion and to provide clarity. In actual situations, assessment, resuscitation or treatment, reevaluation, and diagnosis may occur simultaneously, but priorities should not change.

A. Primary Survey Assessment of ABCDEs

1. Airway with cervical spine protection
2. Breathing with management of life-threatening chest injuries
3. Circulation with control of hemorrhage
4. Disability: Brief neurologic evaluation with intracranial mass lesion recognition
5. Exposure/Environment: Completely undress the patient, but prevent hypothermia

B. Resuscitation

1. Oxygenation and ventilation
2. Shock management, intravenous lines, and Ringer's lactate
3. The management of life-threatening problems identified in the primary survey is continued.

C. Adjuncts to Primary Survey and Resuscitation

1. Monitoring
   a. Arterial blood gas analysis and ventilatory rate
   b. Patient's exhaled CO_2 with an appropriate monitoring device
   c. Electrocardiograph
   d. Patient's hourly urinary output
   e. Pulse oximetry
   f. Blood pressure

2. Urinary and gastric catheters

3. X rays and diagnostic studies
   a. Chest X ray
   b. Pelvis X ray
   c. Cervical spine X ray
   d. DPL or FAST

D. Reassess the Patient's ABCDEs and Consider Need for Transfer

E. Secondary Survey, Total Patient Evaluation: Physical Examination and History

1. Head and skull
2. Maxillofacial
3. Neck
4. Chest
5. Abdomen
6. Perineum/rectum/vagina
7. Musculoskeletal
8. Complete neurologic examination
9. Tubes and fingers in every orifice

F. Adjuncts to the Secondary Survey

Specialized diagnostic procedures that are utilized to confirm suspected injury should only be performed after the patient's life-threatening injuries have been identified and managed and the patient's hemodynamic and ventilation status has returned to normal.

1. Computerized tomography
2. Contrast X ray studies
3. Extremity X rays
4. Endoscopy and ultrasonography

G. Patient Reevaluation

Reevaluate the patient, noting, reporting, and documenting any changes in the patient's condition and responses to resuscitative efforts. Judicious use of analgesics is required. Continuous monitoring of the patient's vital signs and urinary output is essential.

H. Transfer

If the patient's injuries exceed the institution's immediate treatment capabilities, the process of transferring the patient is initiated as soon as the need is identified. The referring doctor and receiving doctor should communicate directly. Transfer personnel should be adequately skilled to administer the required patient care en route. Delay in transferring the patient to a facility with a higher level of care may significantly increase the patient's risk of mortality.

I. Definitive Care

Definitive care begins after identifying the patient's injuries, managing life-threatening problems, and obtaining special studies. The principles of definitive care, associated with the major trauma entities, were described previously in this document.

APPENDICES

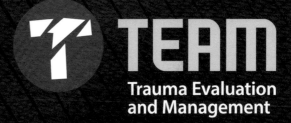

team teach

work cooperat

single group o

team·work (tē

which individ

ciency; coord

with a team

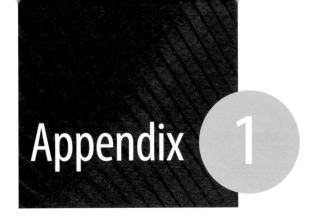

Appendix 1

Glossary of Frequently Confused Terms

TERM	DEFINITION
Cardiac Tamponade	Cardiac tamponade occurs when blood from an injured heart, great vessel, or pericardial vessel fills the pericardial sac. The human pericardial sac is a fixed fibrous structure, and only a relatively small amount of blood is required to restrict cardiac activity and interfere with cardiac filling. Cardiac tamponade most commonly results from penetrating injuries, but blunt injuries also may cause this condition.
Flail Chest	A flail chest occurs when a segment of the chest wall does not have bony continuity with the rest of the thoracic cage. This condition usually results from trauma associated with multiple rib fractures, that is, two or more ribs fractured in two or more places. The presence of a flail chest segment results in severe disruption of normal chest wall movement with underlying lung contusion.
Massive Hemothorax	Massive hemothorax results from a rapid accumulation of more than 1,500 mL of blood in the chest cavity. It is most commonly caused by a penetrating wound that disrupts the systemic or hilar vessels, but it also may be the result of blunt trauma. Massive hemothorax can significantly compromise respiratory efforts by compressing the lung and decreasing ventilation, but more dramatically presents as hypotension and shock.
Open Pneumothorax *(Sucking chest wound)*	When a large defect of the chest wall occurs and remains open, it results in an open pneumothorax or sucking chest wound. Equilibration between intrathoracic pressure and atmospheric pressure is immediate. If the opening in the chest wall is approximately two-thirds the diameter of the trachea, air passes preferentially through the chest defect with each respiratory effort, because air tends to follow the path of least resistance through the large chest-wall defect. Effective ventilation is thereby impaired, leading to hypoxia and hypercarbia.
Neurogenic Shock	Neurogenic shock results from loss of sympathetically mediated peripheral vasomotor tone and reflex tachycardia secondary to disruption of sympathetic nerve fibers in the spinal cord. The result is hypotension, usually without tachycardia and with peripheral vasodilatation, manifested by warm extremities.
Shock	Shock is an abnormality of the circulatory system that results in inadequate organ perfusion and tissue oxygenation.
Simple Pneumothorax	Pneumothorax results from air entering the pleural space between the visceral and parietal pleurae. Both penetrating and nonpenetrating trauma may cause this injury. Air in the pleural space collapses lung tissue, which causes a ventilation/perfusion defect because the blood perfusing the nonventilated area is not oxygenated.
Spinal Shock	Spinal shock is a neurologic phenomenon resulting from complete cessation of all spinal cord function below the level of the spinal cord injury. The result is flaccidity, areflexia, and loss of sensation. These findings are usually temporary, but of variable duration.
Tension Pneumothorax	A tension pneumothorax develops when a "one-way-valve" air leak occurs either from the lung or through the chest wall. Air is forced into the thoracic cavity without any means of escape, completely collapsing the affected lung. The mediastinum is displaced to the opposite side, decreasing venous return to the heart and compressing the opposite lung.

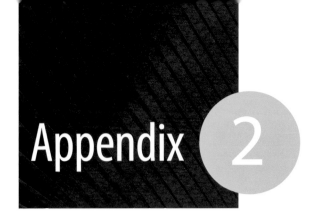

Appendix 2

Prehospital Triage Decision Scheme

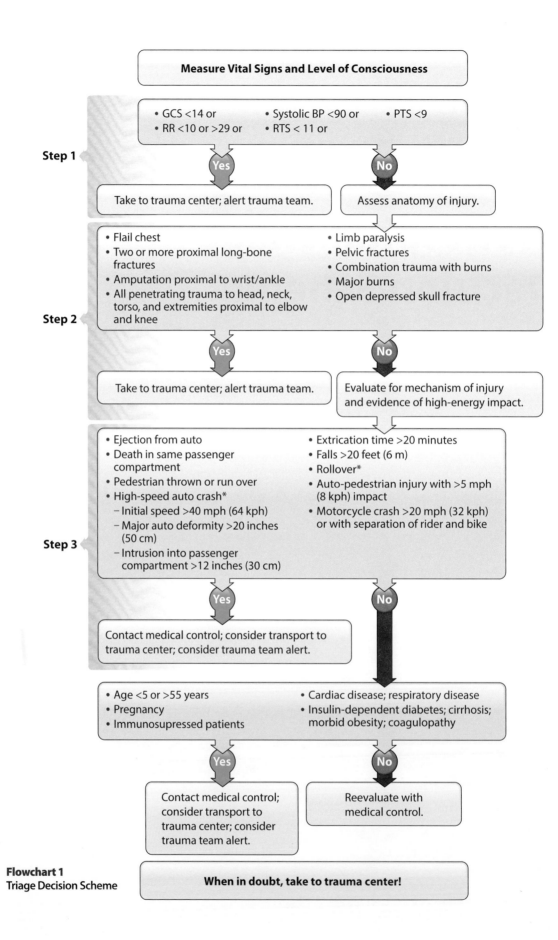

Measure Vital Signs and Level of Consciousness

Step 1

- GCS <14 or
- RR <10 or >29 or
- Systolic BP <90 or
- RTS < 11 or
- PTS <9

Yes → Take to trauma center; alert trauma team.

No → Assess anatomy of injury.

Step 2

- Flail chest
- Two or more proximal long-bone fractures
- Amputation proximal to wrist/ankle
- All penetrating trauma to head, neck, torso, and extremities proximal to elbow and knee

- Limb paralysis
- Pelvic fractures
- Combination trauma with burns
- Major burns
- Open depressed skull fracture

Yes → Take to trauma center; alert trauma team.

No → Evaluate for mechanism of injury and evidence of high-energy impact.

Step 3

- Ejection from auto
- Death in same passenger compartment
- Pedestrian thrown or run over
- High-speed auto crash*
  - Initial speed >40 mph (64 kph)
  - Major auto deformity >20 inches (50 cm)
  - Intrusion into passenger compartment >12 inches (30 cm)

- Extrication time >20 minutes
- Falls >20 feet (6 m)
- Rollover*
- Auto-pedestrian injury with >5 mph (8 kph) impact
- Motorcycle crash >20 mph (32 kph) or with separation of rider and bike

Yes → Contact medical control; consider transport to trauma center; consider trauma team alert.

No ↓

- Age <5 or >55 years
- Pregnancy
- Immunosupressed patients

- Cardiac disease; respiratory disease
- Insulin-dependent diabetes; cirrhosis; morbid obesity; coagulopathy

Yes → Contact medical control; consider transport to trauma center; consider trauma team alert.

No → Reevaluate with medical control.

Flowchart 1
Triage Decision Scheme

When in doubt, take to trauma center!

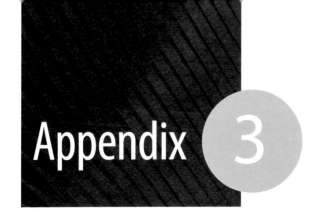

Appendix 3

Revised and Pediatric Trauma Scores

Revised And Pediatric Trauma Scores

Correct triage is essential to effective function of regional trauma systems. Overtriage inundates trauma centers with minimally injured patients, who then impede care for severely injured patients. Undertriage can produce inadequate initial care and may cause preventable morbidity and mortality. Unfortunately, the perfect triage tool does not exist.

Experience with adult trauma scoring systems illustrates this problem by the multiplicity of scoring systems that have been proposed over the last decade. None of these scoring protocols is universally accepted as a completely effective triage tool. At present, most adult trauma surgeons utilize the Revised Trauma Score (RTS) as a triage tool and the weighted variation of this score as a predictor of potential mortality. This score is based totally on physiologic derangement on initial evaluation and entails a categorization of blood pressure, respiratory rate, and the Glasgow Coma Scale. (See Table 1, Revised Trauma Score.)

Application of these three components to the pediatric population is difficult and inconsistent. Respiratory rate is often inaccurately measured in the field and does not necessarily reflect respiratory insufficiency in the injured child. The Glasgow Coma Scale is an extremely effective neurologic assessment tool; however, it requires some revision for application to the preverbal child. These problems, in association with the lack of any identification of anatomic injury or quantification of patient size, undermine the applicability of the Revised Trauma Score to effective triage of the injured child. For these reasons, the Pediatric Trauma Score (PTS) was developed. The PTS is the sum of the severity grade of each category and has been demonstrated to predict potential for death and severe disability reliably. (See Table 2, Pediatric Trauma Score.)

Size is a major consideration for the infant-toddler group, in which mortality from injury is the highest. **Airway** is assessed not just as a function, but also as a descriptor of what care is required to provide adequate management. **Systolic blood pressure** assessment primarily identifies those children in whom evolving preventable shock may occur (50 to 90 mm Hg systolic blood pressure [+1]). Regardless of size, a child whose systolic blood pressure is below 50 mm Hg (-1) is in obvious jeopardy. On the other hand, a child whose systolic pressure exceeds 90 mm Hg (+2) probably falls into a better outcome category than a child with even a slight degree of hypotension.

Level of consciousness is the most important factor in the initial assessment of the central nervous system. Because children frequently lose consciousness transiently during injury, the "obtunded" (+1) grade is given to any child who loses consciousness, no matter how fleeting the loss. This grade identifies a patient who may have sustained a head injury with potentially fatal—but often treatable—intracranial sequelae.

Skeletal injury is a component of the PTS because of its high incidence in the pediatric population and its potential contribution to mortality. Finally, **cutaneous injury,** both as an adjunct to common pediatric injury patterns and as an injury category that includes penetrating wounds, is considered in the computed PTS.

The PTS serves as a simple checklist, ensuring that all components critical to initial assessment of the injured child have been considered. It is useful for paramedics in the field, as well as for doctors in facilities other than pediatric trauma units. As a predictor of injury, the PTS has a statistically significant inverse relationship with the Injury Severity Score (ISS) and mortality. Analysis of this relationship has identified a threshold PTS of eight, below which all injured children should be triaged to an appropriate pediatric trauma center. Children with a PTS of more than eight have the highest potential for preventable mortality, morbidity, and disability. Conversely, children with a PTS of eight have an identifiable mortality risk. According to the National Pediatric Trauma Registry statistics, these children represent approximately 25 percent of all pediatric trauma victims, clearly requiring the most aggressive monitoring and observation.

Recent studies comparing the PTS with the RTS have identified similar performances of both scores in predicting potential for mortality. Unfortunately, the RTS produces unacceptable levels of undertriage, which is an inadequate trade-off for its greater simplicity. Perhaps more importantly, however, the PTS's function as an initial assessment checklist requires that each of the factors that may contribute to death or disability be considered during initial evaluation and become a source of concern for those individuals responsible for the initial assessment and management of the injured child.

TABLE 1: REVISED TRAUMA SCORE				
ASSESSMENT COMPONENT	VARIABLES	SCORE	START OF TRANSPORT	END OF TRANSPORT
A. Respiratory Rate (breaths/minute)	10–29 >29 6–9 1–5 0	4 3 2 1 0	_____	_____
B. Systolic Blood Pressure (mm Hg)	>89 76–89 50–75 1–49 0	4 3 2 1 0	_____	_____
C. Glasgow Coma Scale Score Conversion C = D + E1+ F (adult) C = D + E2+ F (pediatric)	13–15 9–12 6–8 4–5 <4	4 3 2 1 0	_____	_____
D. Eye Opening	Spontaneous To voice To pain None	4 3 2 1	_____	_____
E^1 Verbal Response, Adult	Oriented Confused Inappropriate words Incomprehensible words None	5 4 3 2 1	_____	_____
E^2 Verbal Response, Pediatric	Appropriate Cries, consolable Persistently irritable Restless, agitated None	5 4 3 2 1	_____	_____
F. Motor Response	Obeys commands Localizes pain Withdraws (pain) Flexion (pain) Extension (pain) None	6 5 4 3 2 1	_____	_____
Glasgow Coma Scale Score (Total = D + E1 or E2+ F)			_____	_____
Revised Trauma Score (Total = A + B + C)			_____	_____

Adapted with permission from Champion HR, Sacco WJ, Copes WS, et al: A revision of the Trauma Score. *Journal of Trauma.* 1989; 29(5):624.

TABLE 2: PEDIATRIC TRAUMA SCORE			
ASSESSMENT COMPONENT	**SCORE**		
	+2	**+1**	**-1**
Weight	>20 kg (>44 lb)	10–20 kg (22–44 lb)	<10 kg (<22 lb)
Airway	Normal	Oral or nasal airway; oxygen	Intubated, cricothyroidotomy, tracheostomy
Systolic Blood Pressure	>90 mm Hg; good peripheral pulses, perfusion	50–90 mm Hg; carotid/femoral pulses palpable	<50 mm Hg; weak or no pulses
Level of Consciousness	Awake	Obtunded or any LOC[1]	Coma; unresponsive
Fracture	None seen or suspected	Single, closed	Open or multiple
Cutaneous	None visible	Contusion, abrasion; laceration <7 cm; not through fascia	Tissue loss; any GSW/SW[2] through fascia
Totals:			

[1] Loss of consciousness
[2] GSW = Gunshot wound; SW = Stab wound

Adapted with permission from Tepas JJ, Mollitt DL, Talbert JL, et al: The pediatric trauma score as a predictor of injury severity in the injured child. *Journal of Pediatric Surgery* 1987; 22(l):l5.

TABLE 3: PEDIATRIC VERBAL SCORE	
VERBAL RESPONSE	**V-SCORE**
Appropriate words or social smile, fixes and follows	5
Cries, but consolable	4
Persistently irritable	3
Restless, agitated	2
None	1

Notes:

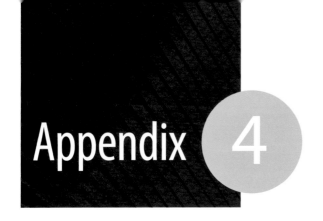

Appendix 4

Mechanisms of Automotive Injury and Related, Suspected Injury Patterns

TABLE 1: MECHANISMS OF AUTOMOTIVE INJURY AND RELATED, SUSPECTED INJURY PATTERNS

MECHANISMS OF INJURY	RELATED, SUSPECTED INJURY PATTERNS
Frontal impact, automobile collision • Bent steering wheel • Knee imprint, dashboard • Bull's eye fracture, windscreen	• Head and brain injury • Maxillofacial injury • Cervical spine fractures • Anterior flail chest • Myocardial contusion • Pneumothorax • Traumatic aortic disruption • Fractured spleen or liver • Posterior fracture/dislocation of hip, knee
Side impact, automobile collision	• Contralateral neck sprain • Cervical spine fracture • Lateral flail chest • Pneumothorax • Traumatic aortic disruption • Diaphragmatic rupture • Fractured spleen/liver, kidney, depending on side of impact • Fractured pelvis or acetabulum
Rear impact, automobile collision	• Cervical spine injury • Soft-tissue injury to the neck
Ejection, vehicle	• Ejection from the vehicle precludes meaningful prediction of injury patterns, but places patient at greater risk from virtually all injury mechanisms • Mortality significantly increases
Motor vehicle, pedestrian	• Head injury • Traumatic aortic disruption • Abdominal visceral injuries • Fractured lower extremities/pelvis

TABLE 2: TOP FIVE INJURY MECHANISMS AND RELATED MORTALITY

	0–5 years	6–10 years	>10 years
Proportion	35%	27%	37%
Mortality	3.1%	2.2%	3.3%
Mechanism	Fall (0.8%) MV (5.3%) Peds (5.3%) Struck (1.9%) Stab (1.0%)	Fall (0.1%) Peds (4.7%) Bike (1.5%) MV (4.6%) Sport (0.7%)	MV (3.9%) Fall (0.5%) Bike (2.2%) GSW (9.6%) Sport (0.2%)
Proportion of all injuries	82%	83%	69%

Abbreviations: MV = motor vehicular; peds = pedestrian; stab = stabbing; struck = inadvertently struck by object; GSW = gunshot wound; sport = sports-related. Mortality for each mechanism listed is identified in parentheses beside abbreviation.

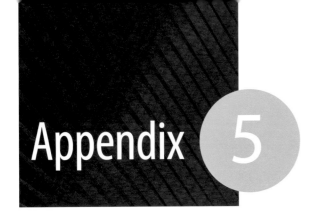

Appendix 5

Guidelines for Managing the Injured Patient

FOR USE IN PRESENTING FOCUSED DISCUSSION CASES AND SIMULATED TRAUMA SCENARIOS

Objectives

Performance at this optional focused discussion on the initial assessment and management of an injured patient allows the participant(s) to practice and demonstrate the following activities in a simulated clinical situation:

1. Communicate and demonstrate to the instructor the systematic initial assessment and management of each patient.

2. Using the primary survey assessment techniques, determine and demonstrate:

   a. Airway patency and cervical spine control
   b. Breathing efficacy
   c. Circulatory status with hemorrhage control
   d. Disability: Neurologic status
   e. Exposure/Environment: Undress the patient, but prevent hypothermia

3. Establish resuscitation (management) priorities in the multiply injured patient based on findings from the primary survey.

4. Demonstrate effective teamwork if multidisciplinary team members are available to assist.

5. Integrate appropriate history taking as an invaluable aid in the assessment of the patient situation.

6. Identify the injury-producing mechanism and discuss the injuries that may exist and/or may be anticipated as a result of the mechanism of injury.

7. Using secondary survey techniques, assess the patient from head to toe.

8. Using the primary and secondary survey techniques, reevaluate the patient's status and response to therapy instituted.

9. Given a series of X rays:

   a. Diagnose fractures

    b.   Differentiate associated injuries

10. Outline the definitive care necessary to stabilize each patient in preparation for possible transport to a trauma center or closest appropriate facility.

11. As referring doctor, communicate with the receiving doctor (instructor) in a logical, sequential manner:

    a.   Patient's history, including mechanism of injury
    b.   Physical findings
    c.   Management instituted
    d.   Patient's response to therapy
    e.   Diagnostic tests performed and results
    f.   Need for transport
    g.   Method of transportation
    h.   Anticipated time of arrival

Note: *Standard precautions are required whenever caring for the trauma patient.*

I. Primary Survey and Resuscitation

The student should (1) outline preparations that must be made to facilitate the rapid progression of assessing and resuscitating the patient, including the utilization of team members; (2) indicate the need to wear appropriate clothing to protect both student and patient from communicable diseases; and (3) indicate that the patient is to be completely undressed, but that hypothermia should be prevented. The following outline serves as a checklist to guide the management of the injured patient.

A. **Airway with Cervical Spine Protection**
  1. Assessment
     a. Ascertain patency; suspect actual or impending airway obstruction in all injured patients.
     b. Rapidly assess for airway obstruction.
     c. Maintain the cervical spine in a neutral position with bimanual immobilization as necessary when establishing an airway.
  2. Management—Establish a patent airway
     a. Perform a chin lift or jaw thrust maneuver.
     b. Clear the airway of foreign bodies.
     c. Administer oxygen-enriched air.
     c. Insert an oropharyngeal or nasopharyngeal airway and avoid prolonged periods of apnea.
     d. If integrity of airway is in doubt, establish a definitive airway by performing
        1) Orotracheal or nasotracheal intubation
        2) Surgical cricothyroidotomy; indicated whenever a definitive airway is needed and nonsurgical attempts at intubation are unsuccessful.
     e. Describe jet insufflation of the airway, noting that it is only a temporary procedure.
     f. Assess and reassess airway patency, endotracheal tube position, and ventilatory effectiveness.
  3. Reinstate immobilization of the cervical spine with appropriate devices after establishing a definitive airway.

B. **Breathing: Ventilation and Oxygenation with Lifethreatening Chest Injury Management**

Thoracic trauma is common in the multiply injured patient and can be associated with life-threatening problems. Patients with thoracic injuries usually can be treated or their conditions temporarily improved or relieved by relatively simple measures, for example, intubation, ventilation, needle decompression, tube thoracostomy, and needle pericardiocentesis. The ability to recognize life-threatening thoracic injuries and skills to perform the necessary procedures can be life saving. An unrecognized tension pneumothorax remains a leading cause of preventable death in patients with thoracic trauma.

  1. Assessment
     a. Expose the neck and chest; ensure immobilization of the patient's head, neck, and entire body.
     b. Determine the rate and depth of respirations.
     c. Inspect and palpate the neck and chest for tracheal deviation, unilateral and bilateral chest movement, use of accessory muscles, and any signs of injury.
     d. Percuss the chest for presence of dullness or hyperresonance.
     e. Auscultate the chest bilaterally.

2. Management—Ventilate and oxygenate
   a. Administer high concentrations of oxygen.
   b. Ventilate with a bag-valve-mask device.
   c. Alleviate tension pneumothorax.
   d. Seal open pneumothorax.
   e. Attach a CO_2-monitoring device to the endotracheal tube.
   f. Attach the patient to a pulse oximeter.

C. Circulation with Hemorrhage Control

Hypovolemia is the cause of shock in most trauma patients. The goal of therapy is prompt restoration of organ perfusion with the delivery of oxygen and substrate to the cell for aerobic metabolism. Management of the patient in shock requires immediate hemorrhage control (in other words, "stop the bleeding"), as well as intravenous fluids and/or blood replacement. Patients who fail to respond to these measures because of continued bleeding usually require operative control of the hemorrhage. Other possible causes of the shock state must be considered in transient responders or nonresponders. The patient's response to initial fluid therapy determines further therapeutic and diagnostic procedures. All patients who manifest signs of hypovolemic shock are potential candidates for surgical exploration. Vasopressors are contraindicated in the management of hypovolemic shock. Central venous pressure measure may be a valuable tool for confirming the volume status and monitoring the rate of fluid administration in selected patients.

1. Assessment
   a. Identify source of external, exsanguinating hemorrhage
   b. Identify potential source(s) of internal hemorrhage
   c. Pulse: Quality, rate, regularity, paradox
   d. Skin color
   e. Blood pressure, time permitting
2. Management—Stop the bleeding, replace the volume
   a. Apply direct pressure to external bleeding site.
   b. Consider presence of internal hemorrhage and potential need for operative intervention, and obtain surgical consultation.
   c. Insert two large-caliber intravenous catheters.
   d. Simultaneously obtain blood for hematologic and chemical analyses, pregnancy test, type and crossmatch, and arterial blood gases.
   e. Initiate IV fluid therapy with warmed Ringer's lactate solution (and blood replacement, if indicated).
   f. Apply the pneumatic antishock garment only to control hemorrhage associated with hypotension in the patient with unstable pelvic fractures.
   g. Prevent hypothermia.

D. Disability: Brief Neurologic Examination

Contact a neurosurgeon as early as possible—preferably even before the patient arrives in the emergency department (patient with suspected or known head/brain injury). If a neurosurgeon is not available at your facility, transfer all moderately or severely head-injured patients to a facility with the resources and capabilities to manage these types of patients.

1. Determine the level of consciousness using the GCS Score.
2. Assess the pupils for size, equality, and reaction.

E. Exposure/Environment: Completely undress the patient, but prevent hypothermia

F. Adjuncts to Primary Survey and Resuscitation

1. Obtain arterial blood gas analysis and ventilatory rate.

2. Monitor the patient's exhaled CO_2 with an appropriate monitoring device.

3. Attach the patient to an ECG monitor.

4. Insert urinary and gastric catheters unless contraindicated, and monitor the patient's hourly urinary output.

5. Consider the need for and obtain (1) an AP chest X ray, (2) an AP pelvis X ray, and (3) a lateral, crosstable cervical spine X ray.

6. Consider the need for and perform DPL or focused assessment sonography in trauma (FAST).

G. Reassess the Patient's ABCDEs and Consider Need for Patient Transfer

Secondary Survey: Reevaluation and Management

A. **AMPLE History and Mechanism of Injury**

1. Obtain AMPLE history from patient, family, or prehospital personnel.

   A **A**llergies

   M **M**edications currently used

   P **P**ast illnesses/**P**regnancy

   L **L**ast meal

   E **E**vents/**E**nvironment related to the injury

2. Obtain history of injury-producing event, identifying injury mechanisms.

B. **Head and Maxillofacial**

Avoid secondary brain injury through vigorous support of the airway, breathing, and circulation. In the comatose patient, secure and maintain the airway by endotracheal intubation. In most ventilated patients, normocapnea is preferred. Aggressive hyperventilation (PCO_2 = 25 to 30 mm Hg) can compromise cerebral perfusion and should only be used for very brief periods when there are signs of impending herniation or acute neurologic deterioration. Otherwise, hyperventilation should be used only in moderation for very brief periods of time to maintaining the PCO_2 at 35 mm Hg or above.

Shock should not be attributed to a head or brain injury. Treat shock aggressively, and look for its cause. Resuscitate the patient with normal saline, Ringer's lactate solution, or a similar isotonic solution without dextrose. Hypotonic solutions should not be used. Avoid both hypovolemia and overhydration. The goal in resuscitating the brain-injured patient is to achieve a euvolemic state. Perform a neurologic examination and determine the patient's GCS Score before paralyzing the patient. Assess the patient for associated injuries.

1. Assessment
   a. Inspect and palpate entire head and face for lacerations, contusions, fractures, and thermal injury.
   b. Reevaluate pupils.
   c. Reevaluate level of consciousness and GCS Score.
   d. Assess eyes for hemorrhage, penetrating injury, visual acuity, dislocation of the lens, and presence of contact lens.
   e. Evaluate cranial nerve function.
   f. Inspect ears and nose for cerebrospinal fluid leakage.
   g. Inspect mouth for evidence of bleeding and cerebrospinal fluid, soft-tissue lacerations, and loose teeth.
   h. Frequently reassess the patient's neurologic status.
   i. Exclude cervical spine injuries radiographically and clinically, and obtain other radiographs/imaging studies as needed.
   j. Contact a neurosurgeon as early as possible.

2. Management

   a. Maintain airway; continue ventilation and oxygenation as indicated.

   b. Control hemorrhage.

   c. Prevent secondary brain injury.

   d. Remove contact lenses.

   e. Transfer all moderately or severely head-/brain-injured patients to a facility with the resources and capabilities to manage these types of patients.

C. Cervical Spine and Neck

Attend to life-threatening injuries while minimizing any movement of the spinal column. Document the patient's history and physical examination to establish a baseline for any changes in the patient's neurologic status. Obtain early consultation with a neurosurgeon and/or orthopaedic surgeon whenever a spinal injury is suspected or detected.

1. Assessment

   a. Inspect for signs of blunt and penetrating injury, tracheal deviation, and use of accessory respiratory muscles.

   b. Palpate for tenderness, deformity, swelling, subcutaneous emphysema, tracheal deviation, and symmetry of pulses.

   c. Auscultate the carotid arteries for bruits.

   d. Obtain a lateral, crosstable cervical spine X ray or CT scan as soon as life-threatening injuries are controlled.

2. Management

   a. Establish and maintain proper inline immobilization and protection of the cervical spine until fractures and spinal cord injuries are excluded.

   b. Transfer patients with vertebral fractures or spinal cord injury to a definitive care facility.

D. Chest

1. Assessment

   a. Inspect the anterior, lateral, and posterior chest wall for signs of blunt and penetrating injury, use of accessory muscles, and bilateral respiratory excursions.

   b. Auscultate the anterior chest wall and posterior bases for bilateral breath sounds and heart sounds.

   c. Palpate the entire chest wall for evidence of blunt and penetrating injury, subcutaneous emphysema, tenderness, and crepitation.

   d. Percuss for evidence of hyperresonance or dullness.

   e. Perform focused subxyphoid pericardial ultrasound examination.

2. Management

   a. Perform needle decompression of the pleural space or tube thoracostomy, as indicated.

   b. Attach the chest tube to an underwater seal drainage device.

   c. Correctly dress an open chest wound.

   d. Perform pericardiocentesis, as indicated.

   e. Transfer the patient to the operating room, if indicated.

E. Abdomen

Early consultation with a surgeon is necessary whenever a patient with possible intraabdominal injuries is brought to the emergency department (casualty room). Once the patient's vital signs are restored, evaluation and management vary depending on the mechanism of injury. The hemodynamically abnormal patient with multiple **blunt injuries** is rapidly assessed for intraabdominal bleeding or contamination from the gastrointestinal tract by performing focused assessment sonography in trauma (FAST) or diagnostic peritoneal lavage (DPL).

The hemodynamically normal patient who is difficult to assess clinically is evaluated by contrast-enhanced CT, with the decision to operate based on the specific organ involved, the magnitude of injury, and clinical judgment.

Patients with **penetrating wounds** in proximity to the abdomen and associated with hypotension, peritonitis, or evisceration require emergent laparotomy (celiotomy). Patients with gunshot wounds that obviously traverse the peritoneal cavity or visceral/vascular area of the retroperitoneum on physical examination or routine X rays also require emergency laparotomy. Asymptomatic patients with anterior abdominal stab wounds that penetrate the fascia or peritoneum on local wound exploration may be evaluated by serial physical examination, DPL, or laparotomy. Asymptomatic patients with flank or back stab wounds that are not obviously superficial are evaluated by serial physical examinations or contrast-enhanced CT, although it may be safer to perform a laparotomy in patients with gunshot wounds to the flank and back.

1. Assessment
    a. Inspect the anterior and posterior abdomen for signs of blunt and penetrating injury, and internal bleeding.
    b. Auscultate for presence/absence of bowel sounds.
    c. Percuss the abdomen to elicit subtle rebound tenderness.
    d. Palpate the abdomen for tenderness, involuntary muscle guarding, unequivocal rebound tenderness, or a gravid uterus.
    e. Obtain a pelvic X ray.
    f. Perform DPL (diagnostic peritoneal lavage)/FAST (focused assessment sonography in trauma) examination, if warranted.
    g. Obtain computerized tomography of the abdomen if the patient is hemodynamically normal.
2. Management
    a. Transfer the patient to the operating room, if indicated.
    b. Apply the pneumatic antishock garment, if indicated for the control of hemorrhage from a pelvic fracture.

F. **Perineum/Rectum/Vagina**
    1. Perineal assessment. Assess for
        a. Contusions and hematomas
        b. Lacerations
        c. Urethral bleeding
    2. Rectal assessment. Assess for
        a. Rectal blood
        b. Anal sphincter tone
        c. Bowel wall integrity
        d. Bony fragments
        e. Prostate position
    3. Vaginal assessment. Assess for
        a. Presence of blood in the vaginal vault
        b. Vaginal lacerations

G. **Musculoskeletal**

The goal of assessing and managing a patient with musculoskeletal trauma is to identify injuries that pose a threat to life and/or limb. Although uncommon, life-threatening musculoskeletal injuries must be properly assessed and managed. Most extremity injuries are appropriately diagnosed and managed during the secondary survey. It is essential to recognize and manage in a timely manner pelvic fractures, arterial injuries, compartment syndrome, open fractures, crush injuries, and fracture-dislocations. Early splinting of fractures and dislocations can prevent serious complications and late sequelae. An awareness of the patient's tetanus status and appropriate treatment are essential and can prevent serious complications.

1. Assessment
    a. Inspect the upper and lower extremities for evidence of blunt and penetrating injury, including contusions, lacerations, and deformity.
    b. Palpate the upper and lower extremities for tenderness, crepitation, abnormal movement, and sensation.
    c. Palpate all peripheral pulses for presence, absence, and equality.
    d. Assess the pelvis for evidence of fracture and associated hemorrhage.
    e. Inspect and palpate the thoracic and lumbar spine by logrolling the patient for evidence of blunt and penetrating injury, including contusions, lacerations, tenderness, deformity, and sensation.
    f. Evaluate the X ray of the pelvis for evidence of a fracture.
    g. Obtain X rays of suspected fracture sites as indicated.

2. Management
    a. Apply and/or readjust appropriate splinting devices for extremity fractures as indicated.
    b. Maintain immobilization of the patient's thoracic and lumbar spine.
    c. Apply the pneumatic antishock garment if indicated for the control of hemorrhage associated with a pelvic fracture, or as a splint to immobilize an extremity injury.
    d. Administer tetanus immunization.
    e. Administer medications, including pain medication, as indicated or as directed by specialist.
    f. Consider the possibility of compartment syndrome.
    g. Perform a complete neurovascular examination of the extremities.

H. **Neurologic**

1. Assessment
    a. Reevaluate the pupils and level of consciousness.
    b. Determine the GCS Score.
    c. Evaluate the upper and lower extremities for motor and sensory functions.
    d. Observe for lateralizing signs.

2. Management
    a. Continue ventilation and oxygenation.
    b. Maintain adequate immobilization of the entire patient.

I. **Adjuncts to the Secondary Survey**

Consider the need for and obtain these diagnostic tests as the patient's condition permits and warrants:

1. Additional spinal X rays
2. CT of the head, chest, abdomen, and/or spine
3. Contrast urography
4. Angiography
5. Extremity X rays
6. Transesophageal ultrasound
7. Bronchoscopy
8. Esophagoscopy

III. Patient Reevaluation

Reevaluate the patient, noting, reporting, and documenting any changes in the patient's condition and responses to resuscitative efforts. Judicious use of analgesics may be employed. Continuous monitoring of vital signs and urinary output is essential.

IV. Transfer To Definitive Care

Outline rationale for patient transfer, transfer procedures, patient's needs during transfer, and need for direct doctor-to-doctor communication.

V. Special Considerations

A. Burn and Cold Injuries

Immediate life-saving measures for the burn patient include the recognition of inhalation injury with early endotracheal intubation and rapid administration of intravenous fluids. The patient's clothing is rapidly removed. The extent and depth of the patient's burns are assessed and identified, and fluids are administered according to the patient's weight and body surface area burned. Peripheral circulation is maintained in circumferential burns by performing an escharotomy as necessary. Burn patients requiring transfer to a burn unit or center are identified.

The cause and severity of cold injuries are determined by obtaining an adequate history and identifying the physical findings, as well as measuring the core temperature with a low-range thermometer (esophageal temperature probe preferred). The patient is immediately removed from the cold environment. The patient's airway, breathing, and circulation are assessed, managed appropriately, and continuously monitored and supported. Rewarming techniques are applied as soon as possible. Patients with hypothermia are not considered dead until rewarming has occurred.

B. Pediatric Trauma

Recognition and management of pediatric injuries require the same astute skills as those required for adults. Unique features of the pediatric trauma patient require special attention to airway anatomy and management, fluid requirements, recognition of CNS injury as well as thoracic and abdominal injuries, diagnosis of extremity fractures, and the recognition of the battered, abused child. Most pediatric trauma results from a blunt mechanism of injury involving the head, mandating an aggressive management approach to the airway and breathing. The child with multiple injuries, including head injury, must be rapidly and appropriately resuscitated to avoid the untoward effects of hypovolemia and secondary brain injury. Early involvement of a qualified surgeon is imperative in the management of the injured child. Nonoperative management of abdominal visceral injuries should be performed only by surgeons in facilities equipped to handle any contingencies in an expeditious manner.

C. **Elder Trauma**

Comorbidities significantly affect the elderly patient's outcome. Early aggressive treatment is essential. All injuries are poorly tolerated due to the lack of cardiorespiratory, renal, hepatic, and metabolic reserves. Volume resuscitation of the elderly injured patient frequently requires close central hemodynamic monitoring.

D. **Trauma in Pregnancy**

Important and predictable anatomic and physiologic changes occur during pregnancy that may influence the evaluation and treatment of the injured pregnant patient. Because of the increased intravascular volume, the pregnant patient can lose a significant amount of her blood volume before tachycardia, hypotension, and other signs of hypovolemia occur. Thus the fetus may be in "in shock" and deprived of vital perfusion while the mother's condition and vital signs appear normal. Positioning the mother with her left side down may take pressure off the vena cava and improve the mother's and the child's hemodynamic status.

Vigorous fluid and blood replacement should be given to correct and prevent maternal as well as fetal hypovolemic shock. Assess specifically for conditions unique to the injured pregnant patient, for example, blunt or penetrating uterine trauma, abruptio placenta, amniotic fluid embolism, isoimmunization, and premature rupture of membranes. Attention also must be directed toward the fetus, the second patient of this unique duo, after its environment is stabilized. The best prevention of fetal demise is early and aggressive maternal resuscitation. A qualified surgeon and obstetrician should be consulted early in the evaluation of the pregnant trauma patient.

Notes:

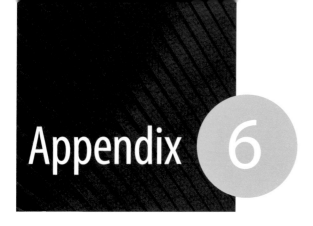

Appendix 6

Slide Handout

No image in the presentation can be used for other purposes without consent from ACS.

The Committee on Trauma Presents

TEAM

Trauma Evaluation and Management:
Early Care of the Injured Patient

Program for Medical Students and Multidisciplinary Team
Members based on the ATLS® Course for Doctors

Slide 1:

_____
_____
_____
_____
_____
_____
_____
_____
_____
_____
_____
_____

Goals/ Principles of Trauma Care

- Rapid, accurate, and physiologic assessment

- Resuscitate, stabilize, and monitor by priority

- Prepare for transfer to definitive care

- Teamwork for optimal, safe patient care

Slide 2:

_____
_____
_____
_____
_____
_____
_____

Illustration: Modified with permission from Trunkey DD. _Scientific American._ 1989; 3:249:28-35.

Objectives

- Describe fundamental principles of initial assessment and management

- Identify correct sequence of management priorities

- Describe appropriate techniques of resuscitation

Slide 3:

_____
_____
_____
_____
_____
_____
_____
_____
_____
_____
_____

Objectives

- Recognize value of patient's history

- Understand importance of injury mechanism

- Identify concepts of teamwork in caring for injured patient

Slide 4:

_____
_____
_____
_____
_____
_____
_____
_____
_____
_____
_____
_____

The Need for Early TEAM

- Leading cause of death in ages 1 through 44
- Disabilities exceed deaths by ratio of 3:1
- Trauma-related costs > $400 billion per year
- Lack of public awareness for injury prevention

Slide 5:

_____
_____
_____
_____
_____
_____
_____
_____
_____
_____

Injury Prevention

 Analyze injury data
 Build local coalitions
 Communicate the problem
 Develop prevention activities
 Evaluate the interventions

Slide 6:

_____
_____
_____
_____
_____
_____
_____
_____
_____
_____

Trimodal Death Distribution

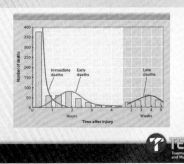

Slide 7:

_____
_____
_____
_____
_____
_____
_____
_____
_____
_____

TEAM Principles

- Treat greatest threat to life first
- Definitive diagnosis less important
- Physiologic approach
- Time is of the essence
- Do no further harm
- Teamwork required for TEAM to succeed

Slide 8:

_____
_____
_____
_____
_____
_____
_____
_____
_____
_____

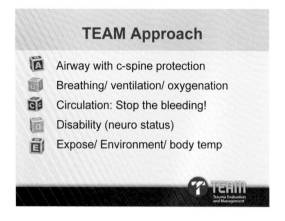

Slide 9:

_____
_____
_____
_____
_____
_____
_____
_____
_____
_____

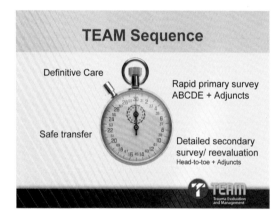

Slide 10:

_____
_____
_____
_____
_____
_____
_____
_____
_____
_____

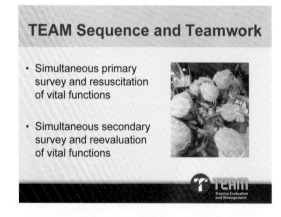

Slide 11:

_____
_____
_____
_____
_____
_____
_____
_____

Photograph courtesy of Charles Aprahamian, MD, FACS.

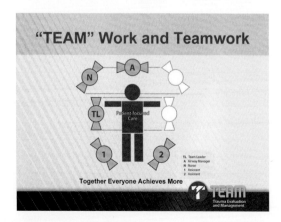

Slide 12:

_____
_____
_____
_____
_____
_____
_____
_____

Illustration courtesy of LTC(P) John Armstrong and MAJ Brad West.

Pre-hospital Preparation

- Closest appropriate facility
- Transport guidelines/ protocols
- On-line medical direction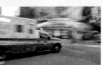
- Mobilization of resources
- Periodic review of care

Slide 13:

_____
_____
_____
_____
_____
_____
_____
_____
_____
_____

In-hospital Preparation

- Preplanning essential
- Team approach
- Trained personnel
- Proper equipment

- Lab / x-ray capabilities
- Standard precautions
- Transfer agreements
- QI Program

Slide 14:

_____
_____
_____
_____
_____
_____
_____
_____
_____
_____

Standard Precautions

- Cap
- Gown
- Gloves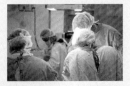
- Mask
- Shoe covers
- Goggles/ face shield

Slide 15:

_____
_____
_____
_____
_____
_____
_____
_____
_____
_____

Triage

- Sorting of patients according to
  - ABCDE's
  - Available resources
  - Other factors, e.g., salvageability

Slide 16:

_____
_____
_____
_____
_____
_____
_____
_____
_____
_____

Primary Survey

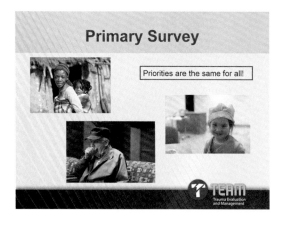

Priorities are the same for all!

Slide 17:

_____

_____

_____

_____

_____

_____

_____

_____

_____

_____

Primary Survey

A Airway / C-spine protection

B Breathing / Life-threatening chest injury

C Circulation / Stop the bleeding

D Disability / Intracranial mass lesion

E Exposure / Environment/ Body temp

Slide 18:

_____

_____

_____

_____

_____

_____

_____

_____

_____

_____

_____

Special Considerations: Children

• Leading cause of death

• Immature, anatomic/ mechanical features

• Vigorous physiologic response

• Limited physiologic reserve

• Outcome depends on early
  aggressive care

Slide 19:

_____

_____

_____

_____

_____

_____

_____

_____

_____

_____

_____

Special Considerations: Children

• Size, dosage, equipment,
  surface area, and psychology

• Airway: Larynx anterior
  and cephalad, short
  tracheal length

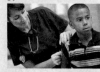

• Breathing: Chest wall pliability,
  mediastinal mobility

Slide 20:

_____

_____

_____

_____

_____

_____

_____

_____

_____

_____

_____

Special Considerations: Children

- Circulation: Vascular access, fluid volume, vital signs, and urinary output

- Neurologic: Vomiting, seizures, and diffuse brain injury

- Musculoskeletal: Immature skeleton, fracture patterns

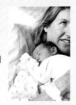

Slide 21:

_____

_____

_____

_____

_____

_____

_____

_____

_____

_____

Special Considerations: Pregnancy

- Anatomic/ physiologic changes modify response to injury

- Need for fetal assessment

- 1st Priority: Maternal resuscitation

- Outcome depends on early, aggressive care

Slide 22:

_____

_____

_____

_____

_____

_____

_____

_____

_____

_____

Special Considerations: Pregnancy

- Gestation and position of uterus
- Physiologic anemia
- ↓ Pco_2
- ↓ Gastric emptying
- Supine hypotension
- Isoimmunization
- Sensitivity of fetus

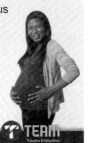

Slide 23:

_____

_____

_____

_____

_____

_____

_____

_____

_____

_____

Special Considerations: Elders

- 5th leading cause of death

- Diminished physiologic reserve and response

- Co-morbidities: Diseases/ Medications

- Outcome depends on early, aggressive care

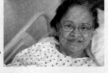

Slide 24:

_____

_____

_____

_____

_____

_____

_____

_____

_____

_____

Primary Survey: Airway

- Assess for airway patency
- Snoring
- Gurgling
- Stridor
- Rocking chest wall motions
- Maxillofacial trauma/ laryngeal injury

CAUTION! C-Spine Injury

Slide 25:

Illustration: Microsoft® ClipArt

Resuscitation: Patent Airway

- Chin lift/ Modified jaw thrust
- Look, listen, feel
- Remove particulate matter
- Definitive airway as necessary
- Reassess frequently

CAUTION! C-Spine Injury

Slide 26:

Illustration: Microsoft® ClipArt

Resuscitation: Assess Breathing

- Chest rise and symmetry
- Air entry
- Rate/ Effort
- Color/ Sensorium

CAUTION! Tension / open pneumothorax

Slide 27:

Resuscitation: Breathing

- Administer supplemental oxygen
- Ventilate as needed
- Tension pneumothorax: Needle decompression
- Open pneumothorax: Occlusive dressing
- Reassess frequently

Slide 28:

Primary Survey: Circulation

- Children
- Elderly
- Athletes
- Pregnancy
- Medications

TEAM
Trauma Evaluation and Management

Slide 29:

_____
_____
_____
_____
_____
_____
_____
_____

Illustration: Microsoft® ClipArt

Primary Survey: Circulation

- Non hemorrhagic shock
  - Cardiac tamponade
  - Tension pneumothorax
  - Neurogenic
  - Septic (late)

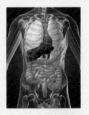

TEAM
Trauma Evaluation and Management

Slide 30:

_____
_____
_____
_____
_____
_____
_____
_____

Illustration: Microsoft® ClipArt

Primary Survey: Circulation

- Assess organ perfusion
  - Level of consciousness
  - Skin color
  - Pulse rate and character

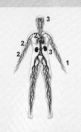

TEAM
Trauma Evaluation and Management

Slide 31:

_____
_____
_____
_____
_____
_____
_____
_____

Illustration: Microsoft® ClipArt

Primary Survey: Circulation

Assess Organ Perfusion
1. Tachycardia
2. Vasoconstriction
2. ↓ Cardiac output
2. Narrow pulse pressure
3. ↓ MAP
3. ↓ Blood flow

TEAM
Trauma Evaluation and Management

Slide 32:

_____
_____
_____
_____
_____
_____
_____
_____
_____

Primary Survey: Circulation

- Children
- Elderly
- Athletes
- Pregnancy
- Medications

Slide 33:

Illustration: Microsoft® ClipArt

Resuscitation: Circulation

Bleeding?

Find it!

- Direct pressure
- Operation
- Avoid blind clamping

Slide 34:

Illustration: Microsoft® ClipArt

Resuscitation: Circulation

- Obtain venous access
- Restore circulating volume
  - Ringer's lactate, 1-2 L
  - PRBCs if transient response or no response
- Reassess frequently

Slide 35:

Resuscitation: Circulation

Table 1
Estimated Fluid and Blood Losses[†]
Based on Patient's Initial Presentation

	Class I	Class II	Class III	Class IV
Blood loss (mL)	Up to 750	750–1500	1500–2000	>2000
Blood loss (% blood volume)	Up to 15%	15%–30%	30%–40%	>40%
Heart rate	<100	>100	>120	>140
Blood pressure	Normal	Normal	Decreased	Decreased
Pulse pressure (mm Hg)	Normal	Decreased	Decreased	Decreased
Respiratory rate	14–20	20–30	30–40	>35
Urine output (mL/hr)	>30	20–30	5–15	Negligible
CNS mental status	Slightly anxious	Mildly anxious	Anxious, confused	Confused, lethargic
Fluid replacement (3:1 rule)	Crystalloid	Crystalloid	Crystalloid and blood	Crystalloid and blood

†For a 70-kg man.

Slide 36:

Resuscitation: Circulation

Consider

- Tension pneumothorax: Needle decompression and tube thoracostomy

- Massive hemothorax: Volume resuscitation and tube thoracostomy

- Cardiac tamponade: Pericardiocentesis and direct operative repair

Slide 37:

_____
_____
_____
_____
_____
_____
_____
_____
_____
_____
_____

Primary Survey: Disability

- Baseline neurologic evaluation

  – Pupillary response
  – Neurosurgical consult as indicated

Observe for neurologic deterioration

Slide 38:

_____
_____
_____
_____
_____
_____
_____
_____

Illustration: Microsoft® ClipArt

Primary Survey: GCS Score

- Eye opening: Range 1-4
- BEST Motor response: Range 1-6
- Verbal response: Range 1-5
- Score = (E + M + V)
- Best score = 15
- Worst score = 3

Slide 39:

_____
_____
_____
_____
_____
_____
_____
_____
_____

Primary Survey: Disability

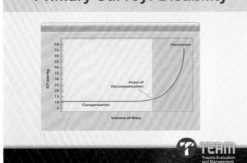

Slide 40:

_____
_____
_____
_____
_____
_____
_____
_____
_____
_____

Primary Survey: Exposure

- Completely undress the patient
- Remove helmet if present
- Look for visible / palpable injuries
- Log roll, protect spine

CAUTION!

Prevent
hypothermia

TEAM
Trauma Evaluation
and Management

Slide 41:

_____
_____
_____
_____
_____
_____
_____
_____
_____
_____

Illustration: Microsoft® ClipArt

Resuscitation: Overview

- If in doubt, establish definitive airway
- Oxygen for all trauma patients
- Chest tube may be definitive for chest injury
- Stop the bleeding!
- 2 large-caliber IVs
- Prevent hypothermia

TEAM
Trauma Evaluation
and Management

Slide 42:

_____
_____
_____
_____
_____
_____
_____
_____
_____
_____
_____

Adjuncts: Urinary Catheter

- Blood?
- Decompress bladder
- Monitor urinary output

CAUTION!

- ❖ Blood at meatus
- ❖ Perineal ecchymosis/ hematoma
- ❖ High-riding prostate

TEAM
Trauma Evaluation
and Management

Slide 43:

_____
_____
_____
_____
_____
_____
_____
_____
_____
_____

Illustration: Microsoft® ClipArt

Adjuncts: Gastric Catheter

- Blood or bile?
- Decompress stomach

CAUTION!

- ❖ CSF rhinorrhea / otorrhea
- ❖ Periorbital ecchymosis
- ❖ Mid-face instability
- ❖ Hemotympanum

TEAM
Trauma Evaluation
and Management

Slide 44:

_____
_____
_____
_____
_____
_____
_____
_____
_____
_____

Illustration: Microsoft® ClipArt

Primary Survey: Adjuncts

Monitoring
- Vital signs
- ABGs
- ECG
- Pulse oximetry
- End-tidal CO_2

Diagnostic Tools
- Chest / pelvis x-ray
- C-spine x-rays when appropriate
- FAST
- DPL

Consider need for transfer

TEAM
Trauma Evaluation and Management

Secondary Survey: Start After

- Primary survey completed

- Resuscitation in process

- ABCDEs reassessed

- Vital functions returning to normal

TEAM
Trauma Evaluation and Management

Secondary Survey: Key Parts

- AMPLE History

- Complete physical exam: Head-to-toe

- Complete neurologic exam

- Special diagnostic tests

- Reevaluation

TEAM
Trauma Evaluation and Management

Secondary Survey: History

A   Allergies
M   Medications
P   Past illnesses / Pregnancy
L   Last meal
E   Events / Environment

TEAM
Trauma Evaluation and Management

Slide 45:

_____
_____
_____
_____
_____
_____
_____
_____
_____
_____
_____

Slide 46:

_____
_____
_____
_____
_____
_____
_____
_____
_____
_____
_____

Slide 47:

_____
_____
_____
_____
_____
_____
_____
_____
_____
_____
_____

Slide 48:

_____
_____
_____
_____
_____
_____
_____
_____
_____
_____
_____

Secondary Survey

Mechanism of Injury

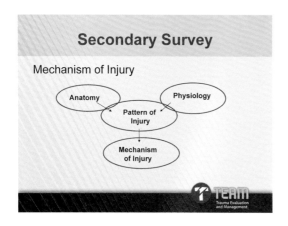

Slide 49:

_____
_____
_____
_____
_____
_____
_____
_____
_____
_____
_____

Burn Injury

- Inhalation injury: Intubate and administer 100% oxygen
- Administer 2 – 4 mL / kg / % BSA burn in 24 hours (+ maintenance in children)
- Monitor urinary output
- Expose and prevent hypothermia
- Chemical burns: Brush and irrigate

Slide 50:

_____
_____
_____
_____
_____
_____
_____
_____
_____
_____
_____

Burn Injury

Rule of Nines

Infant

Adult

Slide 51:

_____
_____
_____
_____
_____
_____
_____

Illustrations used with permission of LifeART Super Anatomy 2 Images and Emergency 3 Images.

Cold Injury

- Frostbite: Rewarm with moist heat (40°C); wait for demarcation

- Hypothermia: Passive or active rewarming

- Monitor: Not dead until warm and dead

Slide 52:

_____
_____
_____
_____
_____
_____
_____
_____
_____
_____

Secondary Survey: Head

- Complete neurologic exam
- GCS Score determination
- Comprehensive eye / ear exam

❖ Unconscious patient
❖ Periorbital edema
❖ Occluded auditory canal

Slide 53:

_____
_____
_____
_____
_____
_____
_____
_____
_____
_____

Secondary Survey: Maxillofacial

- Bony crepitus / instability
- Palpable deformity
- Comprehensive oral / dental exams

❖ Potential airway obstruction
❖ Cribriform plate fracture
❖ Frequently missed injury

Slide 54:

_____
_____
_____
_____
_____
_____
_____

Illustration: Microsoft® ClipArt

Secondary Survey: C-spine

- Palpate for tenderness
- Complete motor / sensory exams
- Reflexes
- C-spine imaging

❖ Injury above clavicles
❖ Altered LOC
❖ Other severe, painful injury

Slide 55:

_____
_____
_____
_____
_____
_____
_____
_____

Illustration: Microsoft® ClipArt

Secondary Survey: Neck

- Blunt vs penetrating
- Airway obstruction, hoarseness
- Crepitus, hematoma, stridor, bruit

❖ Delayed symptoms / signs
❖ Progressive airway obstruction
❖ Occult injuries

Slide 56:

_____
_____
_____
_____
_____
_____
_____
_____

Illustration: Microsoft® ClipArt

Secondary Survey: Chest

- Inspect, auscultate, palpate, percuss
- Reevaluate frequently
- Chest x-rays

CAUTION!
❖ Missed injury
❖ ↑ Chest tube drainage

TEAM
Trauma Evaluation
and Management

Slide 57:

_____
_____
_____
_____
_____
_____
_____
_____
_____

Illustration: Microsoft® ClipArt

Secondary Survey: Abdomen

- Inspect, auscultate, palpate, and percuss
- Reevaluate frequently
- Special studies: FAST, DPL, CT

CAUTION!
❖ Hollow viscus and retroperitoneal injuries
❖ Excessive pelvic manipulation

TEAM
Trauma Evaluation
and Management

Slide 58:

_____
_____
_____
_____
_____
_____
_____
_____
_____

Illustration: Microsoft® ClipArt

Secondary Survey

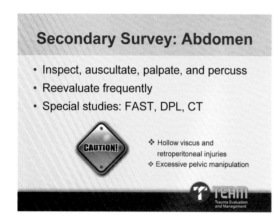

Perineum	Contusions, hematomas, lacerations, urethral blood
Rectum	Sphincter tone, high-riding prostate, pelvic fracture rectal wall integrity, blood
Vagina	Blood, lacerations
	Pregnancy

TEAM
Trauma Evaluation
and Management

Slide 59:

_____
_____
_____
_____
_____
_____
_____
_____
_____

Illustration: Microsoft® ClipArt

Secondary Survey: Musculoskeletal

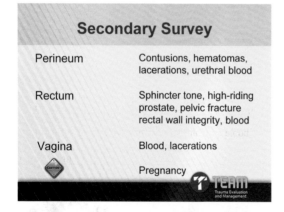

- Potential blood loss
- Limb or life threat (primary survey)
- Missed fractures
- Soft-tissue or ligamentous injury

TEAM
Trauma Evaluation
and Management

Slide 60:

_____
_____
_____
_____
_____
_____
_____
_____
_____

Secondary Survey: Musculoskeletal

- Occult compartment syndrome

  (especially with altered LOC / hypotension)

- Examine patient's back

Slide 61:

_____

_____

_____

_____

_____

_____

_____

_____

_____

_____

Secondary Survey: Pelvis

- Pain on palpation

- Symphysis width ↑

- Leg length unequal

- Instability

- Pelvic x-rays

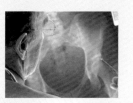

Slide 62:

_____

_____

_____

_____

_____

_____

_____

_____

_____

_____

Pelvic Fracture

- Major source of hemorrhage

- Volume resuscitation

- Reduce pelvic volume

- External fixator

- Angiography / embolization

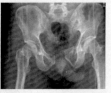

Slide 63:

_____

_____

_____

_____

_____

_____

_____

_____

X-ray courtesy of Ray McGlone, Lancaster Royal Infirmary, UK.

Secondary Survey: CNS

- Frequent reevaluation

- Prevent secondary brain injury

- Imaging as indicated

- Early neurosurgical consultation

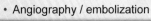

Slide 64:

_____

_____

_____

_____

_____

_____

_____

_____

_____

_____

Secondary Survey: Spine

- Complete motor and sensory exams

- Imaging as indicated

- Maintain inline immobilization

- Early neurosurgical consultation

Slide 65:

_____
_____
_____
_____
_____
_____
_____
_____
_____
_____
_____

Secondary Survey: Neurologic

- Incomplete immobilization

- Subtle ↑ in ICP with manipulation

- Rapid deteriorization

Slide 66:

_____
_____
_____
_____
_____
_____
_____
_____

Illustration: Microsoft® ClipArt

Secondary Survey: Adjuncts

- Blood tests
- Urinalysis
- X- rays
- CT
- Urography
- Angiography

- Ultrasonography
- Echocardiography
- Bronchoscopy
- Esophagoscopy

Do not delay transfer!

Slide 67:

_____
_____
_____
_____
_____
_____
_____
_____
_____
_____

Reevaluation: Missed Injuries

- High index of suspicion

- Frequent reevaluation

- Continuous monitoring

- Rapidly recognize patient deterioration

Slide 68:

_____
_____
_____
_____
_____
_____
_____
_____
_____
_____
_____

Pain Management

- Relieve pain and anxiety as appropriate

- Administer intravenously

- Careful patient monitoring is essential

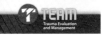

Safe Transfer

When patient's needs exceed institutional resources…

- Use time before transfer for resuscitation
- Do not delay transfer for diagnostic tests
- Physician- to – physician communication

Transfer to Definitive Care

Local facility

Transfer agreements
Local resources

Trauma center

Specialty center

Emergency Preparedness

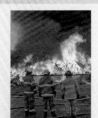

- Simple Plan
- Command structure
- Disaster triage scheme
- Traffic control system

Slide 69:

Slide 70:

Slide 71:

Slide 72:

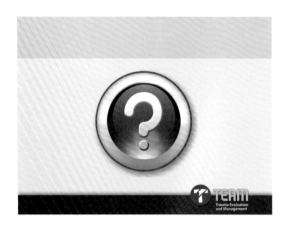

Slide 73:

_____
_____
_____
_____
_____
_____
_____
_____
_____

Illustration: Microsoft® ClipArt

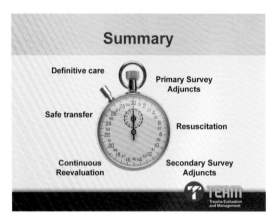

Slide 74:

_____
_____
_____
_____
_____
_____
_____
_____
_____
_____

Slide 75:

_____
_____
_____
_____
_____
_____
_____
_____
_____
_____

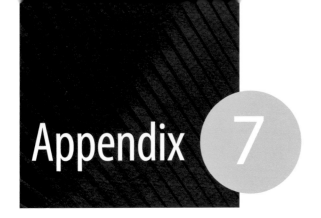

Appendix 7

Program Evaluation Form
by Students

Participants' Evaluation Form

Course Location: _____

Course Date: _____

Your suggestions and criticisms are valuable to us in preparing for future courses and revising the course content. Please assist us by evaluating each session at its completion. Your **overall** rating of each session should include the faculty member's performance as well as the core content (see rating key). Written comments are encouraged and welcomed. It is important that you also respond to the general program items on this form.

Rating: The instructor and session were

Very good = 3	Good = 2	Fair = 1	Poor = 0	Unable to rate = X

SESSION	RATING	COMMENTS
Lecture Content		
• Course content was consistent with the stated objectives • Content was relevant to my educational needs • Instructor rating • Overall session rating		
Video Demonstrations		
• "Bad" Initial Assessment demonstration • "Good" Initial Assessment demonstration • Secondary Survey demonstration		
Focused Discussion Scenarios		
• Instructor rating • Overall session rating		
Simulated Scenario #1		
• Instructor rating • Overall session rating		
Simulated Scenario #2		
• Instructor rating • Overall session rating		
General		
• Discussion time was adequate and enhanced my understanding of the subject • Acquired knowledge will be applied to my practice environment • Room and facilities were appropriate • Program was fair, objective, and unbiased toward any commercial product, institution, or by an individual		

Additional Comments

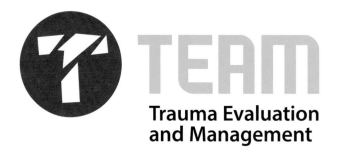

TEAM
Trauma Evaluation
and Management